LOW CARB
DIABETIC
COOKBOOK FOR BEGINNERS

Easy-Made 2500 Days of Delicious, Nutritious Low-Carb & Low-Sugar Recipes for Prediabetes, Type I and Type 2 Diabetes | Includes a 30-Day Meal Plan

DAVID THOMPSON

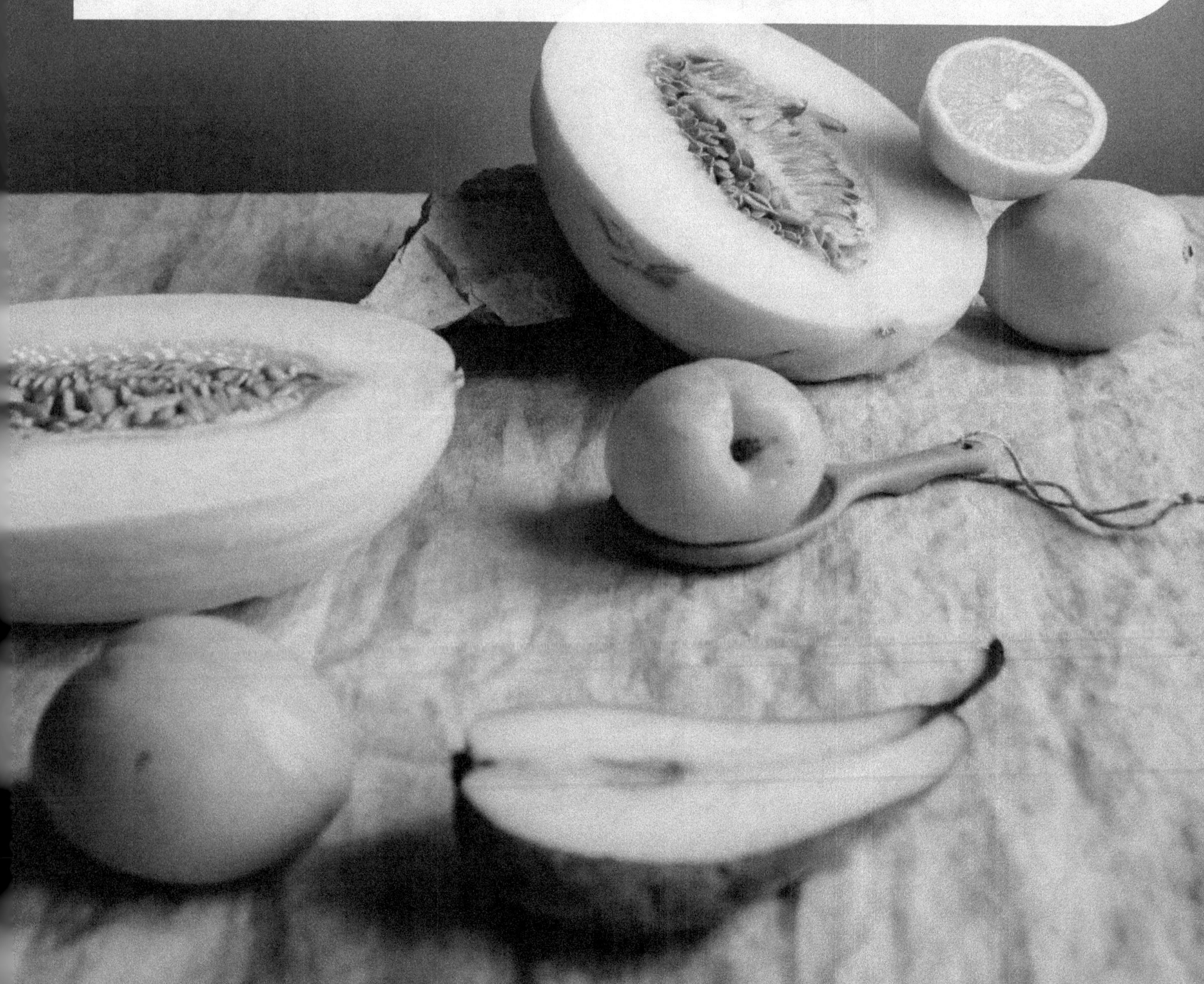

TABLE OF CONTENTS

INTRODUCTION

A low-carb diet, particularly for diabetes management, is more than merely a nutritional adjustment; it is a comprehensive lifestyle change that opens doors to a wealth of health benefits and culinary pleasures. The cornerstone of effective diabetes management lies in understanding the intricate relationship between food and blood sugar levels. A low-carb diet plays an integral role in this equation considering that it provides a scientifically backed, practical approach to keeping glucose levels under control, reducing the requirement for medication, and mitigating the risk of complications linked to diabetes.

The principle behind low-carb eating for diabetes management hinges on the body's metabolism of carbohydrates. Carbohydrates, when broken down during digestion, convert into glucose, leading to a rise in blood sugar levels. For individuals with diabetes, where the body's ability to produce or respond to insulin is impaired, these spikes can be problematic. Reducing carbohydrate intake directly influences lower blood glucose levels, resulting in a more stable and regulated glycemic profile.

Moreover, a low-carb diet's efficacy extends beyond glucose control. Research indicates that such dietary patterns can help lose weight, a crucial aspect of Type 2 diabetes management, by promoting a satiating effect that diminishes hunger and overall intake of calories. The diet also has a positive influence on cardiovascular health indicators, including lowering triglyceride levels and increasing HDL (good) cholesterol levels, addressing two major risk factors for heart disease in individuals with diabetes.

Transitioning to a low-carb lifestyle demands a departure from typical dietary paradigms, steering from refined carbohydrates towards whole, nutrient-dense foods. This change not only ensures blood sugar control, but also enriches the diet with vitamins, minerals, and antioxidants that are necessary for general health. The diet advocates a balanced approach that nourishes the body while delighting the palate, with an emphasis on lean proteins, healthy fats, and low-carb vegetables.

To navigate this journey, it's imperative to acquire an in-depth awareness of food labeling, discerning net carbs, and identifying hidden sugars, ensuring that you make decisions that align with the low-carb principle. In addition, mastering the art of meal planning and preparation is crucial, providing individuals with the ability to maintain dietary adherence without compromising variety or taste.

In the broader context of diabetes management, the integration of physical activity and mindful eating habits with a low-carb diet creates a synergistic effect, boosting insulin sensitivity and fostering a complete sense of well-being. This comprehensive approach stresses the significance of tailored dietary strategies, acknowledging individual preferences, cultural influences, and lifestyle factors to create sustainable, enjoyable eating patterns.

This condition is a path fraught with misconceptions and often, a sense of restriction. However, this book showcases the diversity and complexities of a diet that prioritizes low-carbohydrate ingredients without compromising flavor and satisfaction. Here, we redefine the narrative, demonstrating that a diabetic diet can be as varied and appealing as any other.

At the heart of this cookbook is the belief that a low-carb diet should not be about deprivation but about making informed, smart choices that naturally align with controlling diabetes. The recipes included were curated with careful consideration for their nutritional content, making sure they are low in carbohydrates while rich in proteins and healthy fats. This balance is essential for maintaining stable blood sugar levels, increasing energy, and improving general health while preserving taste and diversity.

Inside, you'll find over 250 recipes in a variety of categories. Each category has been carefully curated to provide you with an extensive range of options, making certain your meals are not only nutritional and diabetic-friendly, but also full of flavor and culinary diversity.

Our 30-Day Meal Plan, an essential component of this cookbook, provides a carefully planned yet adaptable approach to meal planning. It is designed to introduce you to a variety of recipes that can be easily incorporated into your daily routine, allowing you to enjoy a well-balanced diet rich in proteins, healthy fats, and minimal carbohydrates. This meal plan is not solely about following recipes; it's about going on an adventure of discovery, learning to make informed food choices that align with optimal diabetes management.

This cookbook, therefore, is not merely a collection of recipes but a blueprint for a life-changing journey towards health and vitality. It stands as a beacon of hope and empowerment, showcasing that managing diabetes through diet can transcend the realms of necessity into an enriching, life-affirming experience. Through each recipe and every bite, it champions the cause of wellness, proving that with knowledge, commitment, and creativity, living with diabetes can be a journey of discovery, delight, and boundless culinary adventure.

By undertaking this journey, you are taking a significant step toward controlling your diabetes in a way that prioritizes both your health and your enjoyment of eating a meal. Here's to discovering that managing diabetes through nutrition can be a rewarding, pleasant, and genuinely fulfilling experience. Welcome to a new chapter in your dietary journey, one that combines taste, health, and well-being in every bite.

SCROLL down to page 110, scan the QR code to access a trove of exclusive bonuses!

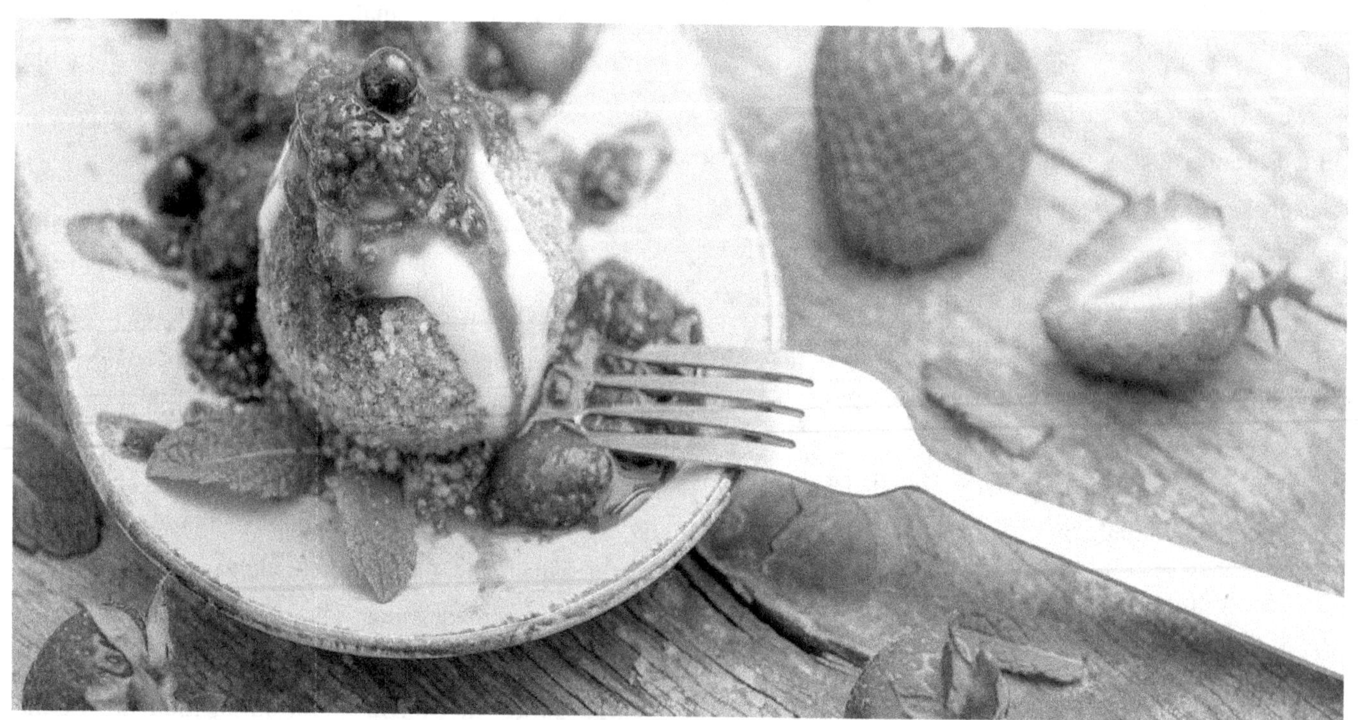

Chapter 1
Understanding Diabetes and Low-Carb Eating

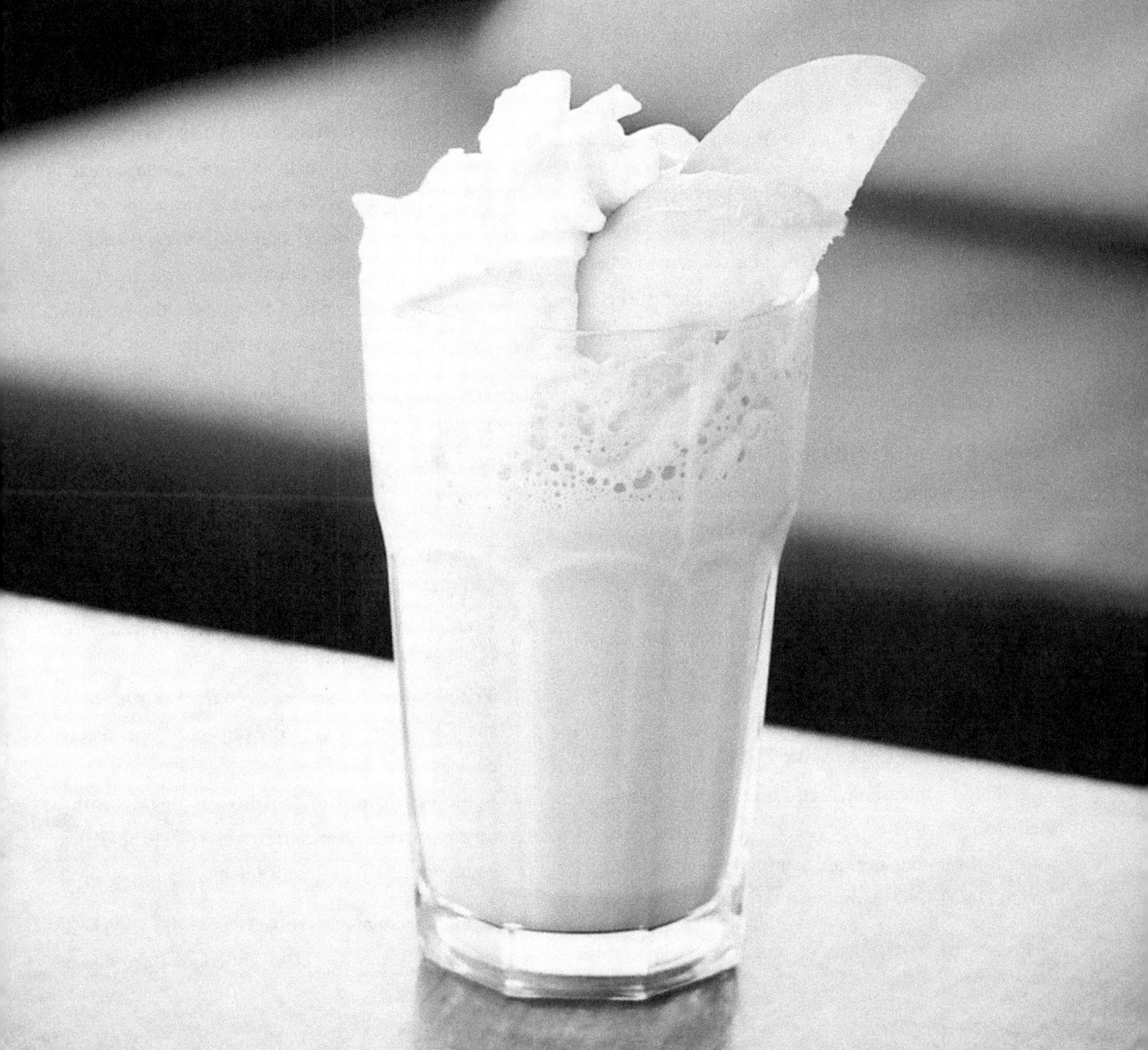

Diabetes represents a long-term health issue marked by elevated glucose, or blood sugar levels. It's imperative for people, particularly those who have recently been diagnosed or are in the process of managing diabetes, to understand the fundamentals of this disease. Such knowledge is the cornerstone for implementing dietary approaches that helps in regulating blood sugar, such as a diet low in carbohydrates.

Types of Diabetes

Type 1 Diabetes: This autoimmune condition results in the body's immune system attacking the insulin-producing cells in the pancreas. Management necessitates consistent insulin administration.

Type 2 Diabetes: This more prevalent form is often associated with lifestyle factors like excess weight and physical inactivity. It develops when the body either resists insulin or doesn't produce sufficient amounts. Management strategies include lifestyle modifications, dietary changes, and sometimes, medications.

Role of Insulin and Glucose

Insulin is a hormone that controls blood sugar by facilitating the entry of glucose's movement into cells for energy. In diabetes, this mechanism is disrupted, leading to elevated blood levels. Without proper management, this can result in severe health issues, such as heart conditions, kidney impairment, and vision problems.

Managing Diabetes with Diet

A diet low in carbohydrates is crucial for managing diabetes, particularly Type 2. This diet reduces carbohydrate consumption to minimize spikes in blood sugar. Here's how to implement it:

Foods to Eat: Focus on non-starchy vegetables (like spinach, kale, and cucumbers), lean proteins (such as chicken breast, fish, and tofu), nuts, seeds, and healthy fats (including avocados and olive oil).

Foods to Avoid: Reduce or eliminate sugary treats, drinks, bread, pasta, rice, and fruits high in carbohydrates.

Benefits of Physical Activity

Regular physical activity improves insulin sensitivity, meaning your cells are better able to use the available sugar in your bloodstream. Activities can vary from gentle activities like walking to more intensive workouts, depending on individual capability and preferences.

Continuous Learning and Adaptation

Continuous education in diabetes management is essential. Recognizing the impact of various foods and exercises on blood sugar helps in making informed daily choices. Regular consultations with healthcare professionals is also critical to monitor the condition and adapt treatment plans as necessary.

Starting a Low-Carb Diet: Practical Steps

Transitioning to a low-carb lifestyle requires understanding and patience. Here are steps to adopt this dietary approach effectively:

1. **Educate Yourself:** Learn about low-carb foods and their health benefits.
2. **Plan Your Meals:** Devise a meal plan that includes appropriate low-carb options.
3. **Track Your Progress:** Keep track of your blood sugar levels to observe the impact of your dietary choices.
4. **Seek Professional Guidance:** Engage with a nutritionist or physician to customize the diet to your specific health requirements.

For individuals embarking on diabetes management, it's essential to understand the disease and the influence of diet on blood sugar. A low-carb diet can be an effective method to manage blood sugar levels. However, it's important to personalize dietary choices to individual health needs and preferences, often with professional guidance, to maintain optimal health and quality of life.

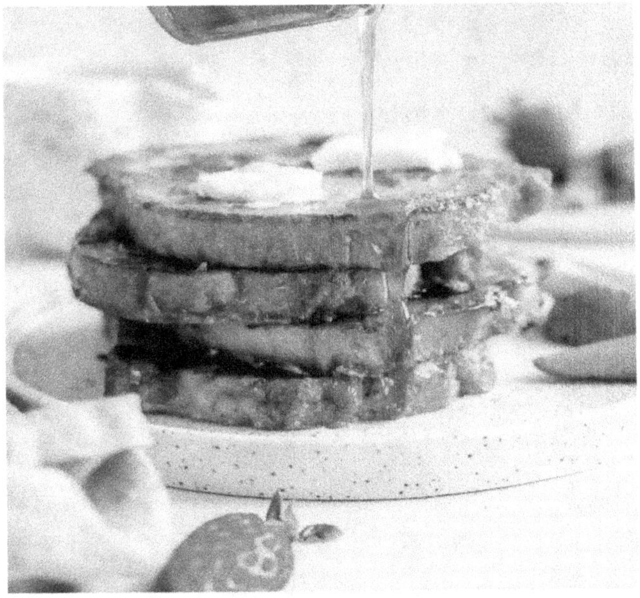

Benefits of a Low-Carb Diet for Diabetics

Embracing a low-carb nutritional regimen is an effective strategy for individuals managing diabetes. This approach focuses on minimizing the intake of carbohydrates to regulate blood sugar levels. This cookbook serves as a guide for those recently diagnosed or struggling with diabetes management, providing insights into the substantial improvements a low-carb diet can bring to their health. In this section, we'll explore the numerous benefits of this dietary plan.

Improved Blood Sugar Control

Stable Blood Sugar Levels: By reducing carbohydrate intake, diabetics can experience fewer spikes in blood sugar levels. Carbohydrates break down into glucose, leading to increases in blood sugar. A low-carb diet limits this reaction, facilitating better glucose control.

Reduced Need for Medication: Consistently low blood sugar levels may reduce the need for insulin or other diabetes medications, under the supervision of a doctor or other medical professional.

Enhanced Weight Management

Promotes Weight Loss: Low-carb diets have been linked to weight loss, a crucial aspect for those with Type 2 diabetes. Weight reduction can improve insulin sensitivity, enabling the body to regulate blood sugar levels more effectively.

Appetite Control: High-fat and high-protein foods often included in low-carb diets can lead to a feeling of fullness, helping to reduce overall calorie intake.

Lower Risk of Cardiovascular Disease

Improved Heart Health Markers: A low-carb diet can lead to improvements in heart health markers, including blood pressure, triglyceride levels, and HDL (good) cholesterol. This is particularly helpful for diabetics, who are at an increased risk of cardiovascular disease.

Enhanced Mental Clarity and Energy

Steady Energy Levels: Fluctuations in blood sugar can lead to energy spikes and crashes. A low-carb diet maintains stable blood sugar, which can contribute to more consistent energy levels throughout the day.

Mental Clarity: Some individuals report improved focus and clarity on a low-carb diet, possibly due to the elimination of sugar spikes that can affect cognitive function.

Potentially Slows the Progression of Diabetes

Long-Term Health Benefits: By effectively managing blood sugar and weight, a diet low in carbohydrates can slow the progression of diabetes, reducing the risk of developing complications related to the disease over time.

Getting Started with a Low-Carb Diet

Adopting a low-carb diet involves understanding which foods to eat and which to avoid, meal planning, and how to monitor and modify carbohydrate consumption depending on personal health goals and responses.

Foods to Include:

- Non-starchy vegetables
- Lean proteins
- Healthy fats
- Nuts and seeds

Foods to Avoid:

- Sugary foods and drinks
- Breads and pastas
- High-carb fruits
- Starchy vegetables

For diabetics, especially those recently diagnosed or seeking to improve their condition, a low-carb diet offers a promising approach to manage and possibly improve their health. Individuals who focus on nutrient-dense, low-carb diets can enjoy a variety of benefits, including better blood sugar control, weight management, reduced risk of cardiovascular disease, and an improved sense of well-being. Consultation with medical professionals is essential to tailor the diet to individual needs, promising both safety and efficacy in diabetes management.

The Glycemic Index Explained

The Glycemic Index (GI) is an important concept for anyone attempting to manage diabetes through diet, especially those just starting out. Understanding the GI can help you make more informed food choices, ultimately leading to better blood sugar control. This section explains the GI, its significance, and how to incorporate it effectively in a diabetic-friendly diet.

What is the glycemic index?

The GI scale classifies carbohydrates on a scale of 0 to 100 based on how much they elevate blood sugar levels after consumption. Foods can be classified as low, medium, or high GI:

Low GI: 55 or below.

Medium GI: 56 to 69

High GI: 70 or above.

Low GI foods cause a slower, more gradual rise in blood sugar levels, while high GI foods induce a rapid increase.

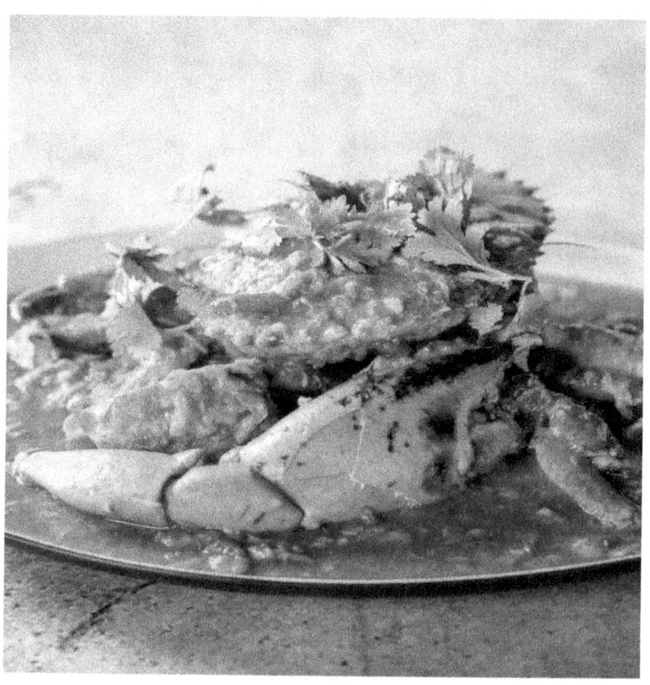

Importance of the Glycemic Index in Diabetes Management

Improved Blood Sugar Control: Integrating more low-GI foods into your diet can help you maintain stable blood sugar levels, which is essential when dealing with diabetes.

Reduced risk of complications: Stable blood sugar levels can lower the risk of diabetes-related complications, such as heart disease, kidney damage, and vision problems.

Weight Management: Low GI diets can help with weight loss and maintenance by promoting a feeling of fullness and reducing appetite.

How to Use the Glycemic Index

Understanding how to utilize the GI efficiently is crucial when incorporating it into a diabetic diet plan.

1. **Choose Low GI Foods:** Opt for foods with a low GI score more often. Examples include non-starchy vegetables, fruits (such as apples and oranges), legumes, and whole grains.
2. **Balance Meals:** Combine high GI foods with low GI foods to balance the meal and minimize blood sugar spikes.
3. **Consider portion sizes:** Even low-GI food, when consumed in large quantities, can affect blood sugar levels. Paying attention to portion sizes is key.

Incorporating Glycemic Index into Your Diet

Here are some practical strategies to include the GI in your daily meal planning:

1. **Educate Yourself:** Learn the GI values of common foods. There are numerous resources and charts available for reference.
2. **Plan your meals:** Include a variety of low and medium GI foods in your meals to maintain a balanced diet.
3. **Monitor Your Blood Sugar:** Keep track of your blood sugar levels to figure out how different GI foods affect you. Individual responses can differ.

Foods and Their Glycemic Index

Low GI Foods: Most non-starchy vegetables, legumes, whole grains, nuts, and some fruits.

Medium GI Foods: Some fruits (like melons and pineapples), sweet potatoes, and whole wheat products.

High GI Foods: White bread, white rice, many cereals, and sugary snacks.

The Glycemic Index is an effective tool for managing diabetes through diet. Individuals with diabetes can better regulate their blood sugar levels, manage their weight, and minimize the risk of complications by choosing foods with lower GI scores. This cookbook aims to provide the knowledge and recipes required to properly implement the GI, hence promoting a healthier lifestyle for those with diabetes.

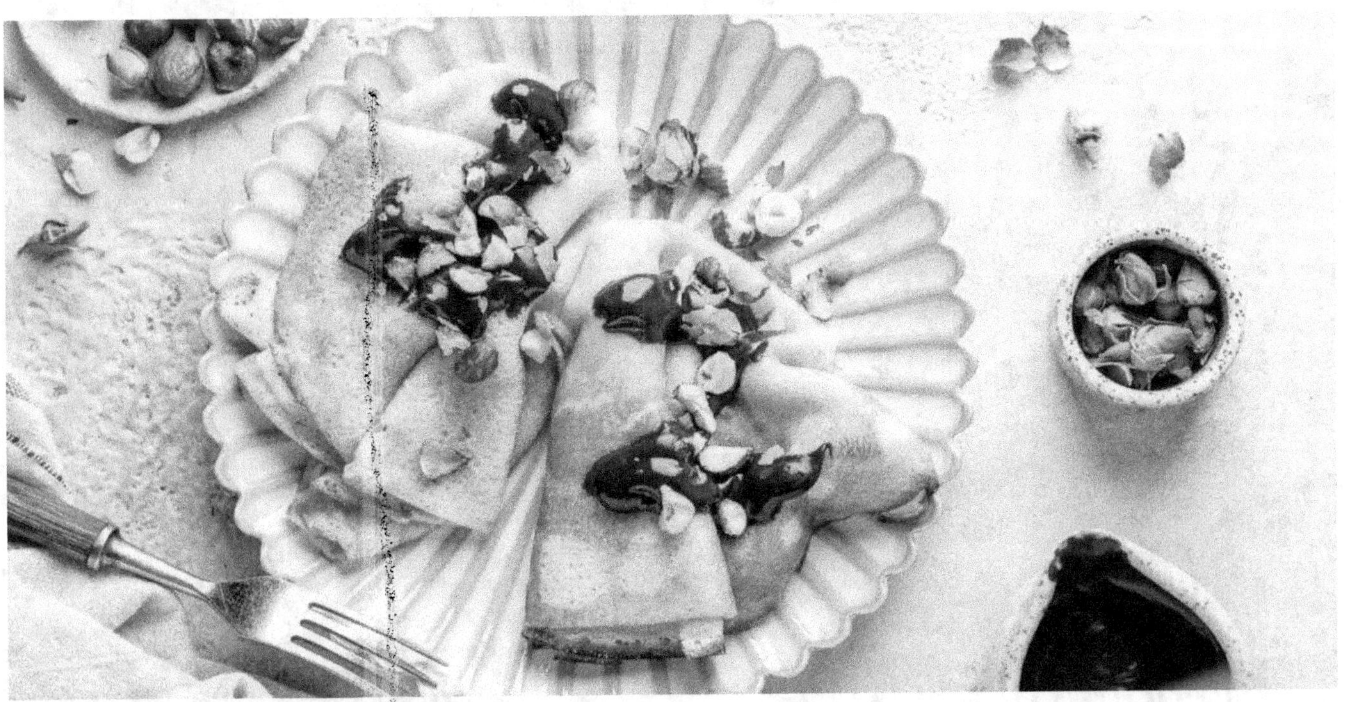

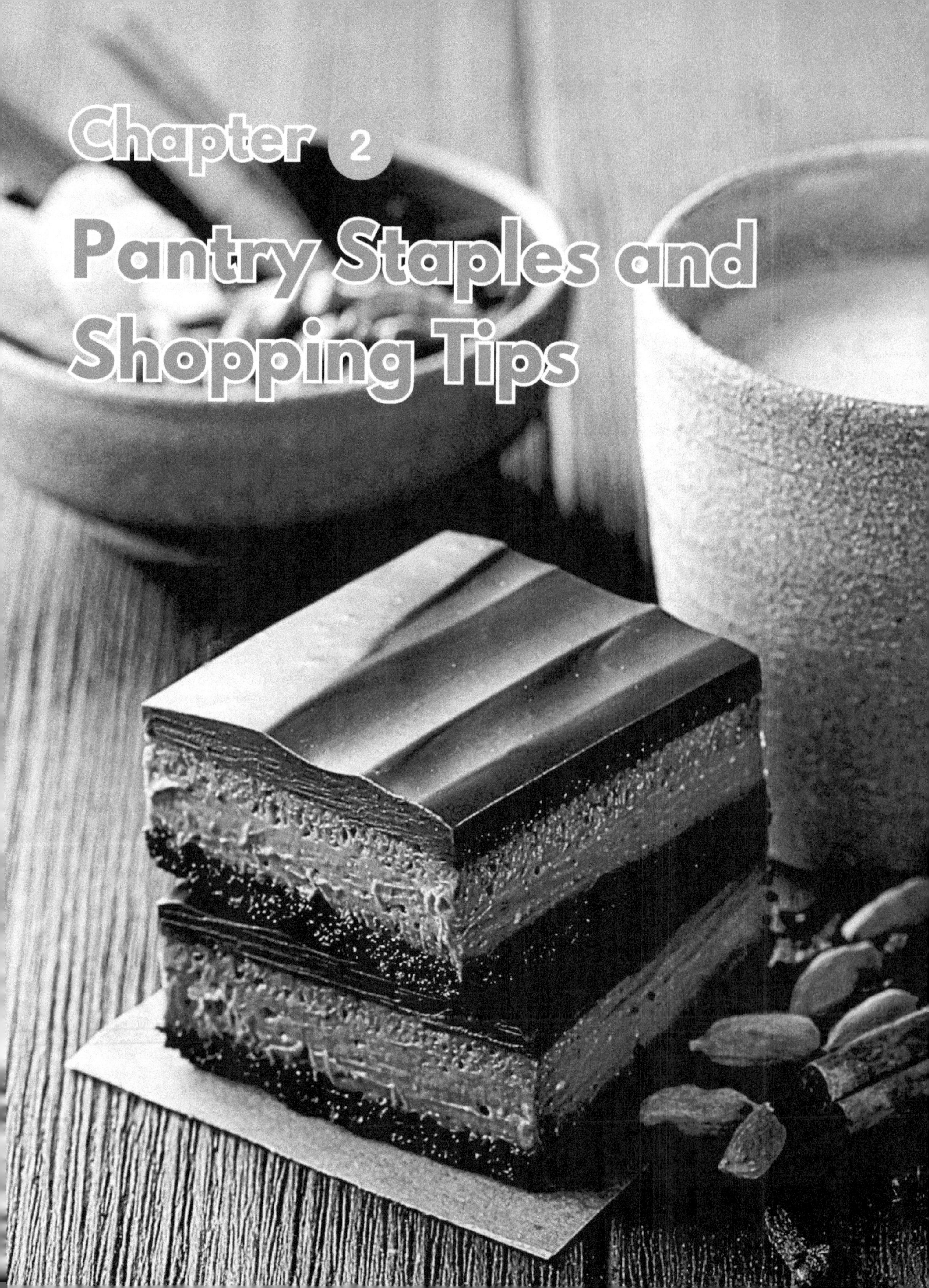

Chapter 2
Pantry Staples and
Shopping Tips

<u>Essential Low-Carb Ingredients</u>

Starting a low-carb diet, especially for people with diabetes, requires rethinking the pantry and grocery list. This cookbook focuses on ingredients that are essential for preparing delicious, nutritious meals that support blood sugar control. Below, we'll look at the fundamental low-carb ingredients that should become kitchen staples.

Proteins

Lean Meats: Chicken, turkey, and lean cuts of beef and pork provide high-quality protein without the carbs. They are adaptable and can be used in a variety of dishes.

Fish and seafood: Salmon, trout, and shrimp are high in omega-3 fatty acids and ideal for a low-carb diet.

Eggs: Highly nutritious and versatile, eggs can be prepared in a variety of ways, making them a suitable low-carb staple.

Healthy fats

Avocados: Packed with fiber and healthy fats, avocados are great for adding creaminess to recipes without adding carbohydrates.

Nuts and Seeds: Almonds, walnuts, chia seeds, and flaxseeds are low in carbs but high in fiber and healthy fats.

Olive Oil and Coconut Oil: Ideal for cooking and dressing, these oils are abundant in healthy fats and contain zero carbs.

Low-carb vegetables

Leafy Greens: Spinach, kale, and other leafy greens are rich in nutrients and very low in carbohydrates.

Cruciferous Vegetables: Broccoli, cauliflower, and Brussels sprouts supply fiber, vitamins, and minerals while containing little carbs.

Other Vegetables: Zucchini, bell peppers, and asparagus are also excellent choices for adding variety and nutrition without many carbs.

Dairy: Hard cheeses such as cheddar, parmesan, and mozzarella are low in carbohydrates and can enhance the flavor and richness of meals.

Greek yogurt and cottage cheese: Choose full-fat versions for lower carbs and a rich source of protein.

Butter and Cream: Used in moderation, these can add flavor and help you feel satisfied on a low-carb diet.

Low-carb fruits

Berries: Strawberries, raspberries, and blueberries can be enjoyed in limited amounts due to their lower carb content compared to other fruits.

Tomatoes: Technically classified as a fruit, tomatoes can add flavor to a number of recipes without contributing an excessive amount of carbohydrates.

Avocados: Though mentioned under healthy fats, avocados deserve a second nod here for their adaptability to low-carb diets.

Pantry staples

Almond and Coconut Flour: These are excellent flour substitutes for baking and cooking.

Sweeteners: Stevia, erythritol, and monk fruit sweeteners are natural options that do not affect blood sugar levels.

Spices and Herbs: Fresh or dried, they add flavor without adding dietary carbs.

Tips for Using These Ingredients

Creativity in the Kitchen: Experiment with different combinations of these ingredients to make meals interesting and delightful.

Meal Planning: To keep your low-carb diet on

track, build your meals around these essentials.

Portion Control: While these ingredients are low in carbohydrates, portion size is still important, particularly for weight management and blood sugar control.

Stocking up on these essential low-carb ingredients will enable you to prepare tasty and nutritious meals that are appropriate for a low-carb, diabetic-friendly diet. You can accomplish your health goals by focusing on high-quality proteins, healthy fats, low-carb vegetables and fruits, and smart pantry staples.

Reading Food Labels

Understanding how to read food labels is an essential skill for anyone on a low-carb diet, particularly those managing diabetes. This section aims to demystify the process, focusing on key aspects that impact blood sugar levels and general well-being.

The Essentials of Food Labels

When purchasing a food item, the label is the most useful tool for determining its nutritional value. Starting with the serving size, this figure is essential because all nutritional information provided is based on this quantity. It's easy to ignore, but understanding how many servings you're actually consuming can have a significant effect on your carb intake and blood sugar management.

Next, pay close attention to the total carbohydrates section. This number comprises sugars, starches, and dietary fiber. Since fiber does not increase blood sugar levels like other kinds of carbohydrates, subtracting fiber from total carbs gives you net carbs, a more precise indicator of a food's impact on blood sugar.

Sugars, both natural and artificial, are also classified as carbohydrates. Added sugars are particularly important to avoid for individuals with diabetes as they can quickly elevate blood sugar levels. The ingredient listings are equally informative. Ingredients are listed in order of quantity, so the first few ingredients make up the bulk of the food. Keep an eye out for different names for sugar, like high fructose corn syrup, which can have an effect on your blood sugar.

Nutritional claims on packaging can sometimes be misleading. Phrases like "low-carb" or "sugar-free" may not necessarily indicate that the product is suitable for your diet. Always verify the nutritional information to ensure it fits within your dietary regimen.

Understanding fats and proteins is also very important. Not all fats are bad, and some, like those from avocados, nuts, and fish, are actually beneficial. Protein content also plays an important role in regulating blood sugar levels.

Practical Tips for Reading Labels

To effectively manage diabetes with a low-carb diet, becoming proficient at reading food labels is important. Here are some practical tips:

1. Start with serving size and servings per container to understand how much you're really eating.
2. Calculate net carbs by subtracting fiber from total carbs, giving you a clearer idea of the food's impact on your blood sugar.
3. Identify any additional sugars in the ingredient list. These can be referred to by a variety of names, so understanding them can help you avoid consuming too much sugar.
4. Do not be swayed by front-of-package marketing. The nutrition facts and ingredient list will always tell you what's real.

For those new to managing diabetes through diet, reading food labels is a mandatory skill. It not only helps in making informed dietary choices, but also in keeping blood sugar levels under control. By focusing on serving size, net carbs, and the types of ingredients, you can manage your diet more effectively, leading to better health outcomes. Remember, the more you practice reading labels, the easier it becomes to select foods that align with your dietary requirements.

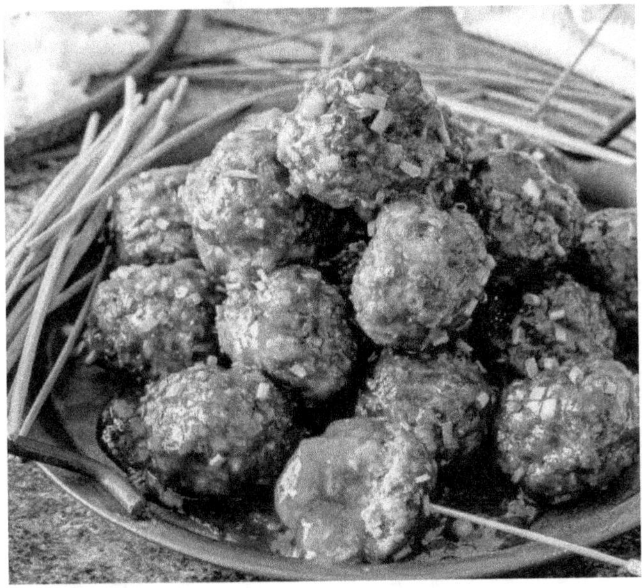

Shopping Tips for Diabetics

Shopping for groceries as a diabetic demands careful consideration to maintain a balanced diet and control blood sugar levels. This section provides valuable insights and ideas to help those new to diabetes make intelligent shopping decisions while navigating the grocery store. These suggestions try to simplify the process, allowing people to enjoy a variety of nutritious and enjoyable meals without compromising their health.

Plan Ahead

The first step towards effective grocery shopping begins at home. Planning is vital. Begin by determining the meals you intend to prepare for the week. This strategy guarantees that you only buy what you need, reducing the temptation to make unhealthy impulsive purchases. Create a precise shopping list that corresponds to your meal plan, with an emphasis on diabetes-friendly foods.

Understand Food Choices

A thorough grasp of which foods are best for controlling diabetes is essential. Your diet should focus on:

- **Low-Carb Vegetables:** Fill your cart with leafy greens, peppers, and other non-starchy vegetables. These are high in nutrients and fiber but low in carbohydrates, which is ideal for blood sugar control.
- **Quality Proteins:** Include lean meats like chicken, turkey, and fish. Plant-based proteins like lentils, beans, and tofu are also excellent choices. These foods help maintain muscle mass and keep you feeling full for a longer period without significantly impacting blood sugar levels.
- **Healthy Fats:** Foods rich in healthy fats, such as avocados, nuts, seeds, and olive oil, can help slow the absorption of glucose into your bloodstream, preventing surges in blood sugar.
- **Whole Grains:** Choose whole grains over processed grains. Quinoa, barley, and oats contain more fiber and have a lower glycemic index than white bread, rice, and pasta.

Reading Labels

Reading nutrition labels is a skill that every diabetic should master. Pay close attention to the total carbohydrate content, including fiber, sugars, and sugar alcohols. Learning to recognize hidden sugars in ingredient lists might also help you avoid food items that cause unexpected blood sugar increase. Remember, the fewer ingredients, and the more recognizable they are, the better.

Shop Smart

When you're in the grocery store, keep the following suggestions in mind:

- **Stick to Your List:** Having a course of action and

sticking to it can help you avoid making unhealthy choices. If it's not on your list, think twice before adding it to your cart.

- **Shop the Perimeter:** Generally, the healthiest foods are often located around the perimeter of the store. This is where you'll find fresh produce, meats, and dairy products. Processed foods, which are generally high in carbohydrates and sugars, can often be found in the aisles.
- **Consider Fresh and Frozen:** Fresh fruits and vegetables are ideal, but frozen variants can be equally nutritious and more convenient. Just make sure they don't contain added sugars or sauces.

Avoid Processed Foods

Processed foods often contain added sugars, unhealthy fats, and calories, which can be detrimental to the management of diabetes. Whenever possible, choose whole or minimally processed foods. This not only supports better blood sugar control, but it also benefits general health.

Embrace Technology

Utilize technology to make shopping easier. Many grocery stores offer applications that can help you organize your shopping trip, access nutritional information, and even clip digital coupons for healthy foods.

Grocery shopping as a diabetic does not have to be difficult. With careful preparation, knowledge of diabetic-friendly meals, and an understanding of how to read food labels, you can make health-conscious decisions. Remember that the items you put in the shopping cart constitute the foundation of your diabetes management plan. By concentrating on nutrient-dense, low-carb options and avoiding processed foods, you can enjoy delicious meals that also help maintain stable blood sugar levels.

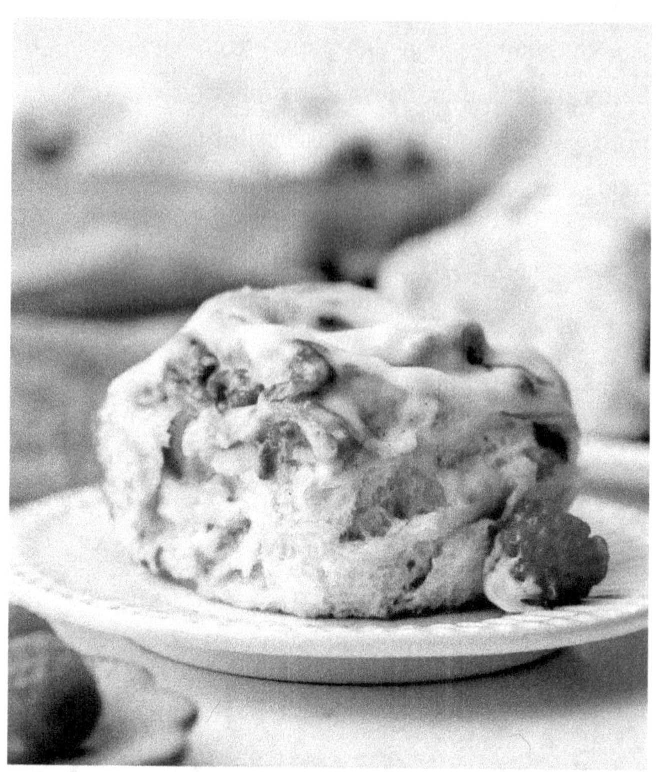

Basic Cooking Techniques for Low-Carb Meals

Mastering basic culinary skills is important for anyone starting a low-carb lifestyle, particularly individuals with diabetes. This section covers several cooking techniques that enhance flavor without adding unnecessary carbohydrates. Using these strategies, you can transform simple ingredients into tasty and nutritious meals. Here's a guide to fundamental cooking techniques for preparing low-carb dishes.

Grilling & Broiling

Grilling and broiling are fantastic ways to prepare meats, seafood, vegetables, and even some fruits, providing depth of flavor and a smoky touch. These methods include cooking food over direct heat, which caramelizes the food's exterior, locking in juices and enhancing natural tastes. These procedures not only minimize the need for added fats, but also assist in preserving the nutritional value of the food. When grilling vegetables or meats, consider marinating them first in herbs and spices combined with olive oil to add extra flavor without carbs.

Roasting

Roasting is the process of cooking food in an oven at a high temperature, which browns the exterior while keeping the interior moist and tender. This approach is suitable for a wide range of vegetables, including Brussels sprouts, cauliflower, and asparagus, as well as meat and poultry. Roasting concentrates flavors and can bring out the natural sweetness in vegetables, making it an excellent way to enjoy the rich flavors of your ingredients without using sugar or other high-carb additives.

Sautéing and Stir-frying

Sautéing and stir-frying involves cooking food quickly in a skillet over medium-high to high heat using only a small amount of fat, such as olive oil or avocado oil. These techniques are ideal for preparing nutritious, crisp-tender vegetables and meats. The rapid cooking time keeps vegetables fresh and rich in nutrients, making this method ideal for stir-fry recipes that combine protein with an assortment of vegetables. Remember to cut your ingredients into small, consistent pieces to ensure even cooking.

Steaming

Steaming is a gentle cooking method that preserves the nutritional value of food by using steam from boiling water to cook it. This method is especially useful for vegetables as it preserves their color, texture, and nutritional integrity without the need for additional fats or oils. Steaming can also be used to cook fish and poultry, producing moist and tender dishes. To enhance the flavor, consider adding herbs or lemon to the water or steamer basket.

Slow Cooking

Slow cooking is an effortless way to prepare meals, allowing flavors to meld together over several hours. It's especially effective for tougher cuts of meat, as the long, low-temperature cooking process tenderizes the meat while keeping it juicy and rich in flavor. Slow

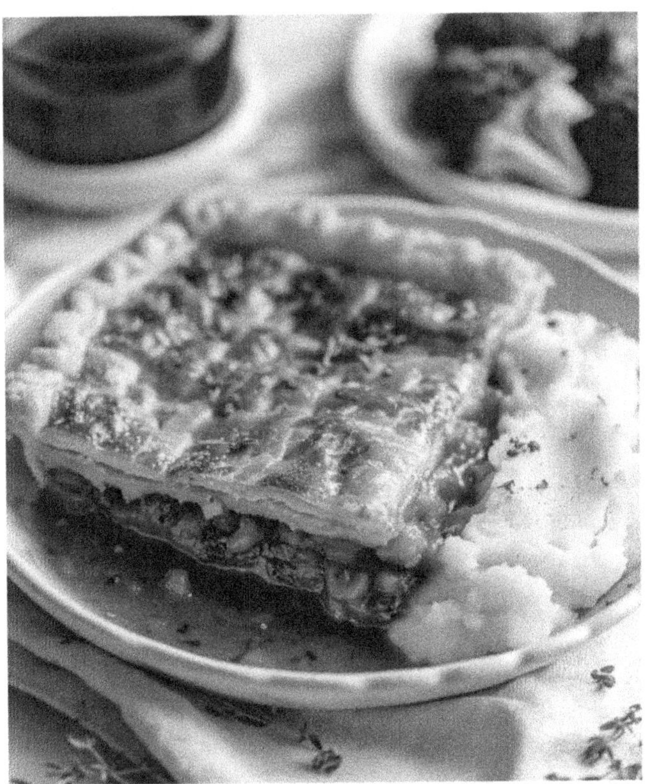

cookers can also be used for preparing a variety of low-carb stews, soups, and casseroles, making it easy to come home to a warm, ready-to-eat meal.

Baking

While conventional baking often involves high-carb ingredients such as flour and sugar, several low-carb substitutes allow you to enjoy baked items. Using almond flour, coconut flour, and natural sweeteners like stevia or erythritol, you can make delightful low-carb versions of your favorite treats. Baking is also an excellent way to make frittatas, quiches, and other egg-based dishes that are nutritious and satisfying.

By mastering these fundamental cooking techniques, you can prepare an extensive selection of low-carb meals that are both satisfying and in line with your nutritional goals. Experimenting with different methods and ingredients will not only add variation to your meals but also guarantee your diet remains enjoyable and sustainable. This cookbook is designed to guide you through this process, offering recipes and suggestions to help you comfortably navigate your low-carb eating habits.

30-DAY MEAL PLAN

DAY	BREAKFAST	LUNCH	SNACK	DINNER
Day 1	Blended Berry Oats	Kale and White Bean Soup	Cheese Crisps with Avocado Dip	Grilled Chicken with Avocado Salsa
Day 2	Greek Yogurt Parfait with Nuts	Portobello Mushroom Steaks	Cucumber and Smoked Salmon Canapés	Spicy Shrimp and Avocado Salad
Day 3	Broccoli and Cheddar Mini Quiches	Mediterranean Chef Salad	Cauliflower Buffalo Bites	Chicken Alfredo Spaghetti Squash
Day 4	Turkey and Spinach Breakfast Sausage Patties	Eggplant and Chickpea Curry	Stuffed Mushrooms with Pesto and Feta	Grilled Tilapia with Mango Salsa
Day 5	Shredded Potato Omelet	Creamy Spinach and Artichoke Casserole	Spinach and Feta Stuffed Portobello Caps	Grilled Chicken and Vegetable Kabobs
Day 6	Flaxseed Meal Porridge	BLT Potato Salad	Baked Parmesan Crisp	Lemon Pepper Tilapia with Broccoli and Carrots
Day 7	Smoked Salmon and Cream Cheese Roll-Ups	Mushroom Hazelnut Rice	Prosciutto-Wrapped Asparagus Spears	Mackerel with Mustard Sauce

DAY	BREAKFAST	LUNCH	SNACK	DINNER
Day 8	Chia Seed Pudding with Berries	Shakshuka with Feta	Avocado and Salsa Stuffed Mini Peppers	Duck Breast with Red Wine Sauce
Day 9	Almond Flour Pancakes	Lentil and Mushroom Stuffed Peppers	Marinated Artichoke Hearts	Beef and Eggplant Lasagna
Day 10	Cottage Cheese and Peach Compote	Low-Carb Ratatouille with Tofu	Spiced Nuts Mix	Balsamic Glazed Chicken Drumsticks
Day 11	Shakshuka with Bell Peppers	Spaghetti Squash and Lentil Bolognese	Zucchini Chips with Herbed Yogurt Dip	Cajun Salmon
Day 12	Raspberry Lemonade Smoothies	Broccoli and Bacon Salad with Cheddar	Olive Tapenade on Cucumber Slices	Pesto Chicken Stuffed Bell Peppers
Day 13	Low-Carb Breakfast Burrito	Vegan Shepherd's Pie with Cauliflower Mash	Deviled Eggs with Smoked Paprika	Shrimp Scampi with Zoodles
Day 14	Coconut Flour Waffles	Mung Bean Sprout Salad	Roasted Garlic and Chive Dip with Vegetable Sticks	Lemon and Herb Roasted Chicken

DAY	BREAKFAST	LUNCH	SNACK	DINNER
Day 15	Spinach and Feta Frittata	Spaghetti Squash Primavera	Jalapeño Poppers Filled with Cream Cheese	Beef and Pepper Fajita Bowls
Day 16	Cucumber and Dill Greek Yogurt Salad	Chia and Flaxseed Oatmeal	Savory Pumpkin Seeds	Sea Bass with Ginger Sauce
Day 17	Egg Muffins with Kale and Tomatoes	Stuffed Cabbage Rolls with Cauliflower Rice	Vegetable Kabobs with Mustard Dip	Chicken Provençal
Day 18	Zucchini and Bell Pepper Omelet	Mediterranean Tuna Salad	Marinated Artichoke Hearts	Baked Halibut with Capers and Olives
Day 19	Pumpkin Seed Granola	Shirataki Rice Pudding	Ricotta and Herb Stuffed Cherry Tomatoes	Zoodles Carbonara
Day 20	Whole-Grain Strawberry Pancakes	Cheesy Zucchini Patties	Stuffed Mushrooms with Pesto and Feta	Cast Iron Hot Chicken
Day 21	Greek Yogurt Parfait with Nuts	Greek Salad with Marinated Feta	Eggplant Rollatini with Ricotta and Spinach	Bacon and Spinach Stuffed Pork Tenderloin

DAY	BREAKFAST	LUNCH	SNACK	DINNER
Day 22	Broccoli Cheese Breakfast Casserole	Thai Red Lentils	Greek Salad Bites	Baked Catfish with Olive Tapenade
Day 23	Bell Pepper and Egg in a Hole	Cauliflower Steaks with Chimichurri Sauce	Spiced Nuts Mix	Turkey Meatloaf with Sun-Dried Tomatoes
Day 24	Bacon and Egg Stuffed Avocado	Low-Carb Refried Beans	Shrimp Cocktail with Sugar-Free Sauce	Lamb Curry with Coconut and Spinach
Day 25	Keto Bagels with Almond Flour	Grilled Salmon Salad with Citrus Dressing	Olive Tapenade on Cucumber Slices	Thai Turkey Lettuce Wraps
Day 26	Cauliflower Hash Browns	Palak Paneer with Tofu	Peanut Butter Protein Bites	Seafood Paella with Cauliflower Rice
Day 27	Almond and Blueberry Smoothie	Hemp Seed Tabouleh	Caprese Skewers with Balsamic Glaze	Lamb Kofta with Tzatziki Sauce
Day 28	Sautéed Greens with Garlic and Poached Eggs	Zucchini Noodle Caprese Salad	Cauliflower Buffalo Bites	Tuna and Avocado Wraps

DAY	BREAKFAST	LUNCH	SNACK	DINNER
Day 29	Mushroom and Spinach Breakfast Skillet	Stuffed Acorn Squash	Chicken Kabobs	Chicken Shawarma Salad
Day 30	Avocado Egg Boats	Roasted Brussels Sprouts with Pecans	Mini Bell Pepper Nachos	Stuffed Bell Peppers with Ground Beef

Note: This 30-Day Meal Plan serves as a guide and inspiration for individuals following a low-carb diet. Please keep in mind that the caloric content of each recipe is only an estimate and may vary depending on portion sizes and specific ingredients used. This plan provides a balanced variety of meals, with an emphasis on proteins, healthy fats, and minimal carbohydrates to support your nutritional goals.

Should the caloric content not fully meet your personal dietary needs, feel free to adjust portion sizes accordingly. Increase or decrease portions to ensure the diet meets your specific health requirements and preferences. Enjoy the flexibility and creativity this plan allows for making nutritious and tasty meals.

For your convenience, we've included a detailed Recipe Index at the end of this book. Here, you'll find the page number for each recipe featured in this meal plan, making it easy to locate each recipe's instructions and caloric information, enabling you in making informed choices that suit your nutritional plan.

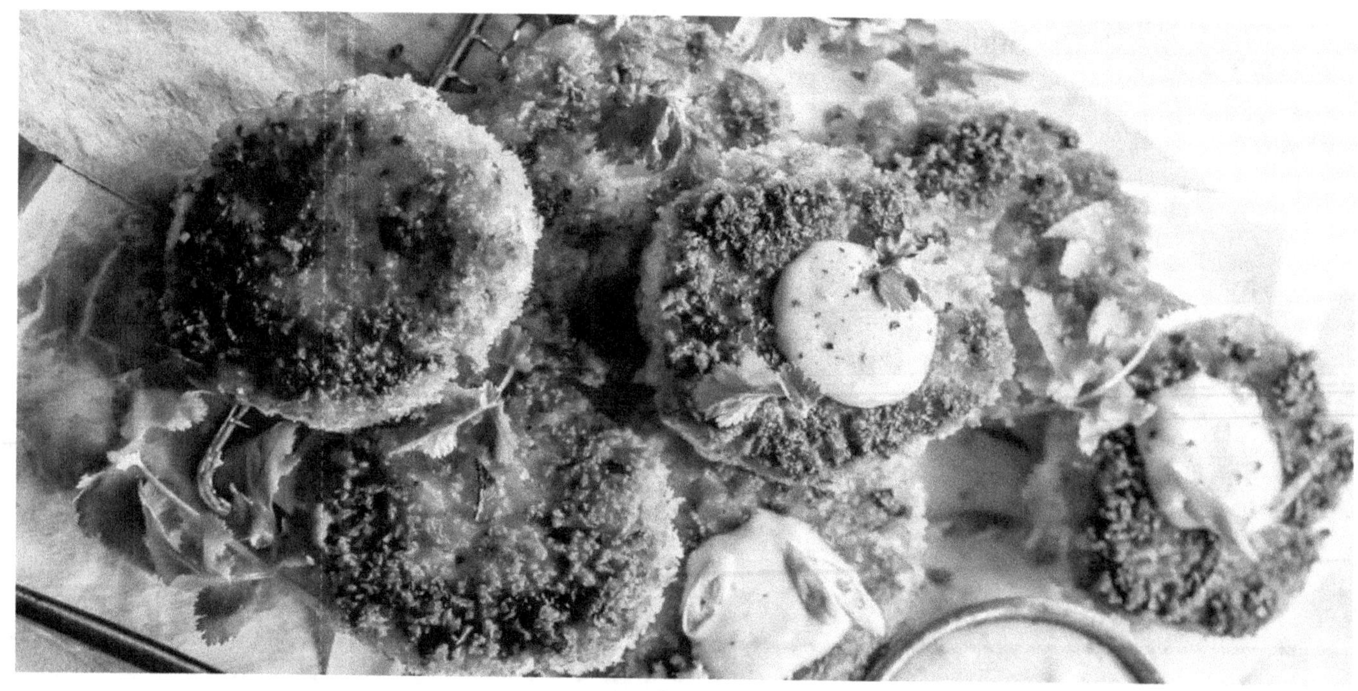

Chapter 3
Breakfasts

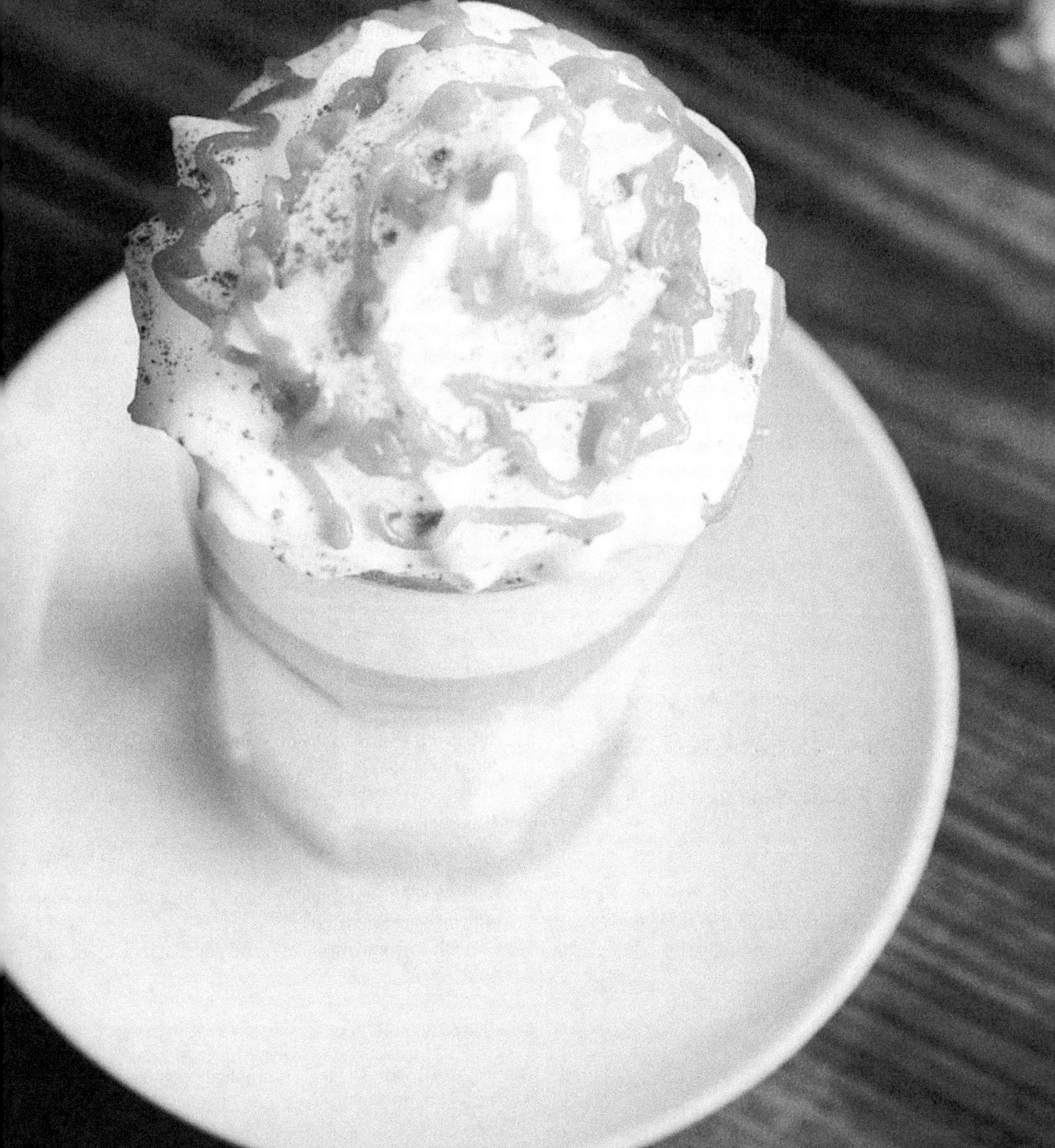

Almond Flour Pancakes

Prep Time: 10 Minutes | **Cook Time:** 15 Minutes | **Serves:** 3

INGREDIENTS:

- 1 cup almond flour
- 3 large eggs
- 1/4 cup water
- 1/4 cup unsweetened almond milk
- 1 tsp vanilla extract
- 1/4 cup tahini
- 1 tbsp erythritol (or sweetener of choice)
- 1/2 tsp baking powder
- Pinch of salt
- Butter or oil for cooking

INSTRUCTIONS:

1. In a mixing bowl, combine almond flour, baking powder, erythritol, and a pinch of salt.
2. In another bowl, whisk together eggs, water, almond milk, and vanilla extract.
3. Mix the wet ingredients into the dry ingredients until a batter is formed.
4. Heat a non-stick skillet over medium heat and add a little butter or oil.
5. Pour 1/4 cup of batter for each pancake, cooking until bubbles form on the surface, then flip and cook until golden brown.
6. Serve warm with your choice of low-carb syrup or fresh berries.

NUTRITIONAL INFORMATION (PER SERVING):

Calories: 280 | Carbs: 6g | Fiber: 3g | Net Carbs: 3g
Protein: 12g

Spinach and Feta Frittata

Prep Time: 10 Minutes | **Cook Time:** 20 Minutes | **Serves:** 4

INGREDIENTS:

- 6 large eggs
- 2 cups fresh spinach, chopped
- 1/2 cup feta cheese, crumbled
- 1/4 cup diced onions
- 1/4 cup heavy cream
- 2 tbsp olive oil
- Salt and pepper to taste

INSTRUCTIONS:

1. Preheat your oven to 375°F (190°C).
2. Heat olive oil in an oven-safe skillet over medium heat. Sauté onions until translucent.
3. Add spinach and cook until wilted.
4. In a bowl, whisk together eggs, heavy cream, salt, and pepper.
5. Pour the egg mixture over the spinach and onions in the skillet. Sprinkle feta cheese on top.
6. Cook without stirring for about 2-3 minutes until the edges start to set.
7. Transfer the skillet to the oven and bake for 15-17 minutes, or until the frittata is set and lightly golden.
8. Let it cool slightly before cutting into wedges and serving.

NUTRITIONAL INFORMATION (PER SERVING):

Calories: 220 | Carbs: 4g | Fiber: 1g | Net Carbs: 3g
Protein: 12g | Fats: 18g

Avocado Egg Boats

Prep Time: 5 Minutes | **Cook Time:** 15 Minutes | **Serves:** 4

INGREDIENTS:

- 2 large avocados, halved and pitted
- 4 small eggs
- Salt and pepper to taste
- 2 tbsp chopped chives or green onions
- 1 tbsp shredded cheese (optional)
- 1/4 tsp paprika (optional)

INSTRUCTIONS:

1. Preheat your oven to 425°F (220°C).
2. Scoop out a little flesh from each avocado half to make room for the eggs.
3. Place the avocado halves in a baking dish, ensuring they are stable.
4. Carefully crack an egg into each avocado half. Season with salt and pepper.
5. Bake for 14-16 minutes, or until the egg whites are set but yolks are still runny.
6. Garnish with chives, cheese, and paprika if desired, and serve warm.

NUTRITIONAL INFORMATION (PER SERVING):

Calories: 180 | Protein: 14g | Carbohydrates: 6g | Fiber: 1g
Fat: 11g | Sodium: 320mg

Cauliflower Hash Browns

Prep Time: 15 Minutes | **Cook Time:** 10 Minutes |
Serves: 4

INGREDIENTS:

- ❖ 1 medium head cauliflower, grated
- ❖ 1 large egg
- ❖ 1/4 cup almond flour
- ❖ 1/4 cup grated Parmesan cheese
- ❖ 1/2 tsp garlic powder
- ❖ Salt and pepper to taste
- ❖ 2 tbsp olive oil for frying

INSTRUCTIONS:

1. Using a clean cloth or cheesecloth, squeeze excess moisture from the grated cauliflower.
2. In a bowl, mix the cauliflower, egg, almond flour, Parmesan, garlic powder, salt, and pepper.
3. Heat olive oil in a skillet over medium heat. Form small patties from the mixture and place them in the skillet.
4. Cook for about 5 minutes per side or until golden brown and crispy. Serve hot.

NUTRITIONAL INFORMATION (PER SERVING):

Calories: 150 | Carbs: 8g | Fiber: 3g | Net Carbs: 5g
Protein: 7g | Fats: 10g

Chia Seed Pudding with Berries

Prep Time: 5 Minutes | **Cook Time:** 0 Minutes |
Serves: 2

INGREDIENTS:

- ❖ 1/4 cup chia seeds
- ❖ 1 cup unsweetened almond milk
- ❖ 1/2 tsp vanilla extract
- ❖ 1 tbsp erythritol or sweetener of choice
- ❖ 1/2 cup mixed berries (fresh or thawed from frozen)

INSTRUCTIONS:

1. In a bowl, whisk together chia seeds, almond milk, vanilla extract, and sweetener until well combined.
2. Let the mixture sit for 5 minutes, then stir again to prevent clumping
3. Cover and refrigerate for at least 2 hours or overnight until it thickens into a pudding consistency.
4. Serve topped with mixed berries.

NUTRITIONAL INFORMATION (PER SERVING):

Calories: 150 | Carbs: 15g | Fiber: 10g | Net Carbs: 5g
Protein: 5g | Fats: 8g

Coconut Flour Waffles

Prep Time: 10 Minutes | **Cook Time:** 15 Minutes |
Serves: 4

INGREDIENTS:

- ❖ 1/2 cup coconut flour
- ❖ 1/4 cup melted butter or coconut oil
- ❖ 4 large eggs
- ❖ 1/2 cup unsweetened almond milk
- ❖ 1 tsp baking powder
- ❖ 1/2 tsp vanilla extract
- ❖ Pinch of salt
- ❖ 1 tbsp erythritol or sweetener of choice

INSTRUCTIONS:

1. Preheat your waffle iron according to the manufacturer's instructions.
2. In a bowl, mix together coconut flour, baking powder, sweetener, and salt.
3. In another bowl, whisk together eggs, melted butter (or coconut oil), almond milk, and vanilla extract.
4. Combine the wet and dry ingredients until a smooth batter is formed.
5. Pour the batter onto the preheated waffle iron and cook according to the waffle iron's instructions, usually about 5 minutes, until golden brown.
6. Serve warm with low-carb syrup or fresh berries.

NUTRITIONAL INFORMATION (PER SERVING):

Calories: 220 | Carbs: 10g | Fiber: 6g | Net Carbs: 1g | Protein: 11g | Fats: 320mg

Greek Yogurt Parfait with Nuts

Prep Time: 5 Minutes | **Cook Time:** 0 Minutes | **Serves:** 2

INGREDIENTS:

- 1 cup full-fat Greek yogurt
- 1/4 cup mixed nuts (almonds, walnuts, pecans), chopped
- 1 tbsp chia seeds
- 1/2 tsp vanilla extract
- 2 tbsp erythritol or sweetener of choice
- 1/4 cup fresh berries (optional)

INSTRUCTIONS:

1. In a bowl, mix the Greek yogurt with vanilla extract and sweetener.
2. In serving glasses or bowls, layer half the yogurt mixture.
3. Add a layer of mixed nuts and chia seeds.
4. Add another layer of the remaining yogurt.
5. Top with fresh berries if desired. Serve immediately or chill for later.

NUTRITIONAL INFORMATION (PER SERVING):

Calories: 220 | Carbs: 10g | Fiber: 3g | Net Carbs: 7g
Protein: 12g | Fats: 15g

Smoked Salmon and Cream Cheese Roll-Ups

Prep Time: 10 Minutes | **Cook Time:** 0 Minutes | **Serves:** 4

INGREDIENTS:

- 8 oz smoked salmon, thinly sliced
- 4 oz cream cheese, softened
- 1 tbsp dill, chopped
- 1 tbsp capers, drained
- 1/4 cup red onion, thinly sliced
- 1 tsp lemon juice
- Pepper to taste

INSTRUCTIONS:

1. Mix the cream cheese with dill, capers, lemon juice, and pepper in a bowl.
2. Lay out slices of smoked salmon on a flat surface.
3. Spread a thin layer of the cream cheese mixture over each slice.
4. Add a few slices of red onion to each piece.
5. Roll up the salmon slices tightly.
6. Cut into bite-sized pieces if desired and serve.

NUTRITIONAL INFORMATION (PER SERVING):

Calories: 180 | Carbs: 2g | Fiber: 0g | Net Carbs: 2g
Protein: 12g | Fats: 14g

Zucchini and Bell Pepper Omelet

Prep Time: 10 Minutes | **Cook Time:** 10 Minutes | **Serves:** 2

INGREDIENTS:

- 4 large eggs
- 1/2 cup zucchini, grated
- 1/2 cup bell pepper, diced
- 1/4 cup onion, diced
- 1/4 cup feta cheese, crumbled
- 2 tbsp olive oil
- Salt and pepper to taste
- Fresh herbs for garnish (optional)

INSTRUCTIONS:

1. Beat the eggs in a bowl, season with salt and pepper.
2. Heat 1 tablespoon of olive oil in a skillet over medium heat. Sauté onion, bell pepper, and zucchini until soft, about 5 minutes.
3. Remove the vegetables and add the remaining olive oil to the skillet.
4. Pour in the eggs, then sprinkle the sautéed vegetables and feta cheese evenly over the top.
5. Cook until the edges start to set, then gently lift the edges and tilt the pan to allow uncooked eggs to flow underneath.
6. Continue cooking until the omelet is set. Fold it in half and slide it onto a plate.
7. Garnish with fresh herbs if desired and serve immediately.

Calories: 300 | Carbs: 6g | Fiber: 1g | Net Carbs: 5g
Protein: 16g | Fats: 24g

Flaxseed Meal Porridge

Prep Time: 5 Minutes | **Cook Time:** 5 Minutes |
Serves: 2

INGREDIENTS:

- 1/2 cup flaxseed meal
- 1 cup unsweetened almond milk
- 1/2 tsp cinnamon
- 1 tbsp erythritol or sweetener of choice
- 1/4 tsp vanilla extract
- Pinch of salt
- 2 tbsp chopped nuts or berries for topping (optional)

INSTRUCTIONS:

1. In a medium-sized saucepan, whisk together the flaxseed meal and almond milk until well combined, ensuring there are no lumps.
2. Place the saucepan over medium heat and add cinnamon, sweetener, vanilla extract, and a pinch of salt to the mixture.
3. Stir the mixture continuously as it heats up. This will prevent it from sticking to the bottom of the pan and ensure even thickening.
4. Once the mixture starts to bubble slightly, reduce the heat to low and continue stirring for another 2-3 minutes until the porridge reaches a creamy consistency.
5. Remove from heat and let it sit for a minute to thicken further.
6. Serve the porridge in bowls and top with your choice of nuts or berries.

NUTRITIONAL INFORMATION (PER SERVING):

Calories: 200 | Carbs: 8g | Fiber: 7g | Net Carbs: 1g
Protein: 6g | Fats: 16g

Blended Berry Oats

Prep Time: 10 Minutes | **Cook Time:** 5 Minutes |
Serves: 2

INGREDIENTS:

- 1/2 cup steel-cut oats or low-carb oat alternative
- 1 cup unsweetened almond milk
- 1/2 cup mixed berries (fresh or frozen)
- 1 tbsp chia seeds
- 1/2 tsp vanilla extract
- 1 tbsp erythritol or sweetener of choice

INSTRUCTIONS:

1. If using steel-cut oats, start by soaking them in almond milk overnight in the refrigerator to soften.
2. In a blender, combine the soaked or alternative oats, almond milk, mixed berries, chia seeds, vanilla extract, and sweetener.
3. Blend the mixture on high until smooth and well combined.
4. Pour the blended mixture into a saucepan and warm over medium heat for about 5 minutes, stirring occasionally to prevent sticking and ensure even warming.
5. Once heated to your liking, remove from heat and pour into serving bowls.
6. You may top with a few extra berries for garnish and added flavor.

NUTRITIONAL INFORMATION (PER SERVING):

Calories: 150 | Carbs: 20g | Fiber: 5g | Net Carbs: 15g
Protein: 5g | Fats: 6g

Cottage Cheese and Peach Compote

Prep Time: 5 Minutes | **Cook Time:** 10 Minutes |
Serves: 2

INGREDIENTS:

- 1 cup cottage cheese
- 2 fresh peaches, pitted and sliced (or equivalent in canned peaches in water, drained)
- 1/2 tsp cinnamon
- 1 tbsp erythritol or sweetener of choice
- 1/4 tsp vanilla extract

1. Begin by preparing the peach compote. In a small saucepan, combine the peach slices, sweetener, cinnamon, vanilla extract, and a small splash of water to help the cooking process.
2. Cook the peach mixture over medium heat, stirring occasionally to prevent sticking and ensure even cooking. The peaches should soften and release their natural juices, creating a syrup-like consistency.
3. Once the peaches have softened and the mixture has thickened slightly (about 8-10 minutes), remove the saucepan from the heat and allow the compote to cool for a few minutes.
4. Place a portion of cottage cheese in each serving bowl.
5. Spoon the warm peach compote over the cottage cheese, allowing the flavors to meld.
6. Serve immediately while the compote is still warm, or chill in the refrigerator if preferred cold.

NUTRITIONAL INFORMATION (PER SERVING):

Calories: 180 | Carbs: 15g | Fiber: 2g | Net Carbs: 30g
Protein: 14g | Fats: 5g

Mushroom and Spinach Breakfast Skillet

Prep Time: 10 Minutes | **Cook Time:** 15 Minutes |
Serves: 2

INGREDIENTS:

- 1 tbsp olive oil
- 1 cup mushrooms, sliced
- 2 cups spinach, fresh
- 4 large eggs
- 1/4 cup feta cheese, crumbled
- Salt and pepper to taste
- 1/2 tsp garlic powder
- Fresh herbs for garnish (optional)

INSTRUCTIONS:

1. Heat olive oil in a large skillet over medium heat. Add mushrooms and sauté until they begin to brown and release their moisture, about 5 minutes.
2. Add spinach to the skillet and cook until it wilts, about 2-3 minutes. Season with salt, pepper, and garlic powder.
3. Make four wells in the vegetable mixture and crack an egg into each well.
4. Cover the skillet with a lid and cook until the egg whites are set but the yolks are still runny, about 5-7 minutes.
5. Sprinkle crumbled feta cheese over the top and garnish with fresh herbs if desired.
6. Serve directly from the skillet, ensuring each portion has an egg.

NUTRITIONAL INFORMATION (PER SERVING):

Calories: 250 | Carbs: 5g | Fiber: 1g | Net Carbs: 4g
Protein: 16g | Fats: 18g

Almond and Blueberry Smoothie

Prep Time: 5 Minutes | **Cook Time:** 0 Minutes |
Serves: 2

INGREDIENTS:

- 1 cup unsweetened almond milk
- 1/2 cup blueberries (fresh or frozen)
- 1/4 cup almond butter
- 1 tbsp chia seeds
- 1/2 tsp vanilla extract
- 1 tbsp erythritol or sweetener of choice
- Ice cubes (optional)

INSTRUCTIONS:

1. Place almond milk, blueberries, almond butter, chia seeds, vanilla extract, sweetener, and ice cubes (if using) in a blender.
2. Blend on high speed until smooth and creamy.
3. Taste and adjust sweetness if necessary.
4. Pour into glasses and serve immediately. You can garnish with a few whole blueberries on top.

NUTRITIONAL INFORMATION (PER SERVING):

Calories: 230 | Carbs: 12g | Fiber: 6g | Net Carbs: 6g
Protein: 7g | Fats: 18g

Prep Time: 15 Minutes | **Cook Time:** 20 Minutes |
Serves: 6

INGREDIENTS:

- 2 cups almond flour
- 1 tbsp baking powder
- 1/2 tsp garlic powder (optional)
- 1/2 tsp onion powder (optional)
- 3 large eggs, divided (2 for dough, 1 beaten for egg wash)
- 2 cups shredded mozzarella cheese
- 2 tbsp cream cheese
- Sesame seeds or poppy seeds for topping (optional)

INSTRUCTIONS:

1. Preheat your oven to 425°F (220°C) and line a baking sheet with parchment paper.
2. In a bowl, mix almond flour, baking powder, garlic powder, and onion powder.
3. In a separate microwave-safe bowl, combine mozzarella and cream cheese. Microwave for 1 minute, stir, and microwave for another 30 seconds until fully melted.
4. Add 2 eggs to the melted cheese mixture and mix well. Then, combine with the almond flour mixture, kneading until a dough forms.
5. Divide the dough into 6 equal portions. Roll each portion into a log and form it into a bagel shape on the prepared baking sheet.
6. Brush each bagel with beaten egg and sprinkle with sesame or poppy seeds.
7. Bake for 12-15 minutes, or until golden brown.
8. Let cool before serving.

NUTRITIONAL INFORMATION (PER SERVING):

Calories: 320 | Carbs: 8g | Fiber: 3g | Net Carbs: 5g
Protein: 18g | Fats: 25g

Bran Apple Muffins

Prep Time: 15 Minutes | **Cook Time:** 20 Minutes |
Serves: 12

INGREDIENTS:

- 1 cup oat bran (use a low-carb alternative if necessary)
- 1/2 cup almond flour
- 1/4 cup flaxseed meal
- 1 tsp baking powder
- 1/2 tsp cinnamon
- 1/4 tsp nutmeg
- Pinch of salt
- 2 large eggs
- 1/4 cup unsweetened applesauce
- 1/4 cup olive oil
- 1/4 cup erythritol or sweetener of choice
- 1 tsp vanilla extract
- 1 medium apple, finely diced

INSTRUCTIONS:

1. Preheat your oven to 350°F (175°C) and line a muffin tin with paper liners or grease well.
2. In a large bowl, combine oat bran, almond flour, flaxseed meal, baking powder, cinnamon, nutmeg, and salt.
3. In another bowl, whisk together eggs, applesauce, olive oil, sweetener, and vanilla extract.
4. Mix the wet ingredients into the dry ingredients until just combined. Fold in the diced apple.
5. Divide the batter evenly among the muffin cups, filling each about 3/4 full.
6. Bake for 18-20 minutes, or until a toothpick inserted into the center comes out clean.
7. Let the muffins cool in the pan for 5 minutes before transferring them to a wire rack to cool completely.

NUTRITIONAL INFORMATION (PER SERVING):

Calories: 140 | Carbs: 12g | Fiber: 4g | Net Carbs: 8g
Protein: 5g | Fats: 9g

Egg Muffins with Kale and Tomatoes

Prep Time: 10 Minutes | **Cook Time:** 20 Minutes |
Serves: 6

INGREDIENTS:

- 6 large eggs
- 1 cup kale, chopped and steamed
- 1/2 cup cherry tomatoes, halved
- 1/4 cup onion, finely diced
- 1/4 cup cheese (optional), shredded
- Salt and pepper to taste

❖ Olive oil or cooking spray for greasing

1. Preheat your oven to 375°F (190°C) and grease a 6-cup muffin tin with olive oil or cooking spray.
2. In a bowl, beat the eggs and season with salt and pepper.
3. Divide the steamed kale, cherry tomatoes, and diced onion evenly among the muffin cups.
4. Pour the beaten eggs over the vegetables, filling each muffin cup about 3/4 full.
5. Sprinkle shredded cheese on top of each muffin cup, if using.
6. Bake for 18-20 minutes, or until the egg muffins are set and lightly golden on top.
7. Allow cooling for a few minutes before removing from the tin. Serve warm.

NUTRITIONAL INFORMATION (PER SERVING):

Calories: 100 | Carbs: 2g | Fiber: 0.5g | Net Carbs: 1.5g
Protein: 8g | Fats: 7g

Ricotta and Lemon Hotcakes

Prep Time: 10 Minutes | **Cook Time:** 15 Minutes |
Serves: 4

INGREDIENTS:

❖ 1 cup almond flour
❖ 1/2 cup ricotta cheese
❖ 2 large eggs
❖ 1/4 cup unsweetened almond milk
❖ 1 tbsp lemon zest
❖ 2 tbsp erythritol or sweetener of choice
❖ 1 tsp baking powder
❖ 1/2 tsp vanilla extract
❖ Butter or oil for cooking

INSTRUCTIONS:

1. In a large bowl, whisk together the almond flour, baking powder, and lemon zest.
2. In another bowl, mix the ricotta cheese, eggs, almond milk, sweetener, and vanilla extract until smooth.
3. Combine the wet and dry ingredients, stirring until a batter is formed.
4. Heat a non-stick skillet or griddle over medium heat and grease lightly with butter or oil.
5. Pour 1/4 cup of batter for each hotcake, cooking until bubbles form on the surface, then flip and cook until golden brown on the other side.
6. Serve warm with a dollop of ricotta or your favorite low-carb syrup.

NUTRITIONAL INFORMATION (PER SERVING):

Calories: 230 | Carbs: 6g | Fiber: 3g | Net Carbs: 3g
Protein: 11g | Fats: 19g

Turkey and Spinach Breakfast Sausage Patties

Prep Time: 15 Minutes | **Cook Time:** 10 Minutes |
Serves: 4

INGREDIENTS:

❖ 1 lb ground turkey
❖ 1 cup spinach, finely chopped
❖ 1/4 cup onion, finely diced
❖ 2 cloves garlic, minced
❖ 1 tsp sage, dried
❖ 1 tsp thyme, dried
❖ 1/2 tsp salt
❖ 1/4 tsp black pepper
❖ 1 tbsp olive oil for cooking

INSTRUCTIONS:

1. In a large bowl, combine ground turkey, chopped spinach, diced onion, minced garlic, sage, thyme, salt, and pepper. Mix thoroughly until all ingredients are well incorporated.
2. Form the mixture into small patties, about 3 inches in diameter.
3. Heat olive oil in a large skillet over medium heat. Place the patties in the skillet and cook for about 4-5 minutes on each side, or until fully cooked through and slightly browned on the outside.
4. Serve hot, either alone or as part of a breakfast plate.

NUTRITIONAL INFORMATION (PER SERVING):

Calories: 100 | Carbs: 2g | Fiber: 0.5g | Net Carbs: 1.5g
Protein: 22g | Fats: 10g

Prep Time: 15 Minutes | **Cook Time:** 10 Minutes |
Serves: 4

INGREDIENTS:

- 4 low-carb tortillas
- 8 eggs
- 1/2 cup cheddar cheese, shredded
- 1 cup spinach, chopped
- 1/4 cup bell peppers, diced
- 1/4 cup onions, diced
- 1/2 cup cooked and crumbled sausage or bacon (optional)
- Salt and pepper to taste
- 1 tbsp olive oil

INSTRUCTIONS:

1. In a skillet, heat olive oil over medium heat. Sauté onions and bell peppers until softened.
2. Beat the eggs in a bowl, season with salt and pepper, and add them to the skillet. Stir in the spinach.
3. Cook, stirring occasionally, until the eggs are scrambled and fully cooked.
4. Warm the low-carb tortillas according to the package instructions.
5. Divide the egg mixture among the tortillas, top with cheese and optional sausage or bacon.
6. Roll up the tortillas to form burritos, folding in the ends to enclose the filling.
7. Serve immediately, or for a crispy exterior, return the burritos to the skillet and cook until golden brown on both sides.

NUTRITIONAL INFORMATION (PER SERVING):

Calories: 300 | Carbs: 15g | Fiber: 9g | Net Carbs: 6g
Protein: 20g | Fats: 18g

Vegetable Frittata

Prep Time: 10 Minutes | **Cook Time:** 25 Minutes |
Serves: 6

INGREDIENTS:

- 1/2 cup heavy cream
- 1 cup zucchini, diced
- 1/2 cup onions, diced
- 1/2 cup tomatoes, diced
- 1 cup bell peppers, diced
- 1/2 cup cheddar cheese, shredded
- 2 tbsp olive oil
- 1/4 cup fresh basil, chopped
- Salt and pepper to taste

INSTRUCTIONS:

1. Preheat your oven to 375°F (190°C).
2. In a large bowl, whisk together eggs, heavy cream, salt, and pepper.
3. Heat olive oil in an oven-safe skillet over medium heat. Sauté onions, bell peppers, and zucchini until softened.
4. Add the tomatoes and cook for an additional 2 minutes.
5. Pour the egg mixture over the vegetables in the skillet. Cook without stirring for 2-3 minutes until the edges begin to set.
6. Sprinkle shredded cheese and chopped basil on top.
7. Transfer the skillet to the oven and bake for 18-20 minutes, or until the frittata is set and the top is lightly golden.
8. Let it cool for a few minutes before slicing and serving.

NUTRITIONAL INFORMATION (PER SERVING):

Calories: 260 | Carbs: 6g | Fiber: 1g | Net Carbs: 5g
Protein: 14g | Fats: 20g

Broccoli and Cheddar Mini Quiches

Prep Time: 15 Minutes | **Cook Time:** 25 Minutes |
Serves: 2 Mini Quiches

INGREDIENTS:

- 2 cups broccoli florets, finely chopped
- 1 cup cheddar cheese, shredded
- 6 large eggs
- 1/2 cup heavy cream
- 1/4 cup onion, finely diced
- Salt and pepper to taste
- Cooking spray or butter for greasing muffin tins

INSTRUCTIONS:

1. Preheat your oven to 350°F (175°C). Grease a 12-cup muffin tin with cooking spray or butter.

2. Steam the broccoli until just tender, then distribute evenly among the muffin cups.
3. Sprinkle the shredded cheddar cheese and diced onion over the broccoli in each cup.
4. In a bowl, whisk together the eggs, heavy cream, salt, and pepper. Pour this mixture into each muffin cup, filling each about 3/4 full.
5. Bake in the preheated oven for 20-25 minutes, or until the quiches are set and lightly golden on top.
6. Let them cool for a few minutes before removing from the muffin tin. Serve warm.

NUTRITIONAL INFORMATION (PER SERVING):

Calories: 120 | Carbs: 2g | Fiber: 0.5g | Net Carbs: 1.5g
Protein: 7g | Fats: 9g

Shakshuka with Bell Peppers

Prep Time: 10 Minutes | **Cook Time:** 25 Minutes |
Serves: 4

INGREDIENTS:

- 1 tbsp olive oil
- 1 large onion, diced
- 1 red bell pepper, diced
- 2 cloves garlic, minced
- 1 tsp paprika
- 1 can (14 oz) diced tomatoes, no sugar added
- Salt and pepper to taste
- 4-6 large eggs
- Fresh parsley or cilantro for garnish
- Feta cheese, crumbled (optional)
- 1/2 tsp cumin

INSTRUCTIONS:

1. Heat olive oil in a large skillet over medium heat. Add onion and bell pepper, cooking until softened, about 5 minutes.
2. Stir in the minced garlic, paprika, and cumin, cooking for another minute until fragrant.
3. Add the diced tomatoes (with juices), salt, and pepper. Simmer the sauce for 10-15 minutes until it thickens slightly.
4. Make wells in the sauce and crack an egg into each well. Cover the skillet and cook until the egg whites are set but the yolks remain runny, about 5-7 minutes.
5. Garnish with fresh parsley or cilantro and crumbled feta cheese if using. Serve directly from the skillet.

NUTRITIONAL INFORMATION (PER SERVING):

Calories: 180 | Carbs: 9g | Fiber: 2g | Net Carbs: 7g
Protein: 10g | Fats: 12g

Raspberry Lemonade Smoothies

Prep Time: 5 Minutes | **Cook Time:** 0 Minute |
Serves: 2

INGREDIENTS:

- 1 cup frozen raspberries
- 1/2 cup unsweetened almond milk
- 1/2 cup Greek yogurt, full-fat
- Juice of 1 lemon
- 2 tbsp erythritol or sweetener of choice
- Ice cubes, as needed

INSTRUCTIONS:

1. In a blender, combine the frozen raspberries, almond milk, Greek yogurt, lemon juice, sweetener, and ice cubes.
2. Blend on high until smooth and creamy. Add more ice if a thicker consistency is desired.
3. Taste and adjust sweetness if necessary. Pour into glasses and serve immediately.

NUTRITIONAL INFORMATION (PER SERVING):

Calories: 100 | Carbs: 8g | Fiber: 4g | Net Carbs: 4g
Protein: 6g | Fats: 4g

Cucumber and Dill Greek Yogurt Salad

Prep Time: 10 Minutes | **Cook Time:** 0 Minute |
Serves: 4

INGREDIENTS:

- 2 large cucumbers, thinly sliced
- 1 cup Greek yogurt, full-fat
- 2 tablespoons fresh dill, chopped
- 1 tablespoon lemon juice

❖ 1 clove garlic, minced
❖ Salt and pepper to taste

INSTRUCTIONS:

1. In a large mixing bowl, combine the sliced cucumbers, Greek yogurt, chopped dill, lemon juice, and minced garlic.
2. Gently toss the ingredients until the cucumbers are well coated with the yogurt mixture.
3. Season with salt and pepper according to taste.
4. Chill in the refrigerator for about 30 minutes before serving to allow the flavors to meld.

NUTRITIONAL INFORMATION (PER SERVING):

Calories: 70 | Carbs: 6g | Fiber: 1g | Net Carbs: 5g
Protein: 4g | Fats: 3g

Pumpkin Seed Granola

Prep Time: 10 Minutes | **Cook Time:** 20 Minutes | **Serves:** 8

INGREDIENTS:

❖ 1 cup pumpkin seeds
❖ 1/2 cup sunflower seeds
❖ 1/2 cup unsweetened shredded coconut
❖ 1/4 cup almond flour
❖ 2 tablespoons chia seeds
❖ 1 teaspoon cinnamon
❖ 1/4 cup melted coconut oil
❖ 1/4 cup sugar-free maple syrup or sweetener of choice
❖ 1 teaspoon vanilla extract

INSTRUCTIONS:

1. Preheat your oven to 300°F (150°C) and line a baking sheet with parchment paper.
2. In a large bowl, mix together the pumpkin seeds, sunflower seeds, shredded coconut, almond flour, chia seeds, and cinnamon.
3. In a separate bowl, whisk together the melted coconut oil, sugar-free maple syrup, and vanilla extract.
4. Pour the wet ingredients over the dry ingredients and stir until everything is well coated.
5. Spread the mixture evenly on the prepared baking sheet and bake for 20 minutes, stirring halfway through, until golden and crispy.
6. Let the granola cool completely before breaking it into clusters.

NUTRITIONAL INFORMATION (PER SERVING):

Calories: 240 | Carbs: 8g | Fiber: 4g | Net Carbs: 4g
Protein: 6g | Fats: 20g

Shredded Potato Omelet

Prep Time: 15 Minutes | **Cook Time:** 10 Minutes | **Serves:** 4

INGREDIENTS:

❖ 2 medium potatoes, peeled and shredded
❖ 6 large eggs
❖ 1/4 cup milk (or almond milk for a lower carb option)
❖ 2 tablespoons olive oil
❖ 1/2 cup shredded cheddar cheese (optional)
❖ 1/4 cup green onions, chopped
❖ Salt and pepper to taste

INSTRUCTIONS:

1. Rinse the shredded potatoes in cold water and squeeze out any excess moisture.
2. Heat olive oil in a large skillet over medium heat. Add the shredded potatoes, season with salt and pepper, and cook until they start to turn golden, about 5 minutes.
3. In a bowl, whisk together the eggs, milk, and additional salt and pepper. Pour this mixture over the potatoes in the skillet.
4. Sprinkle the shredded cheese and green onions on top. Cover and cook over low heat until the eggs are set, about 5 minutes.
5. Cut into wedges and serve warm.

NUTRITIONAL INFORMATION (PER SERVING):

Calories: 220 | Carbs: 15g | Fiber: 2g | Net Carbs: 13g
Protein: 12g | Fats: 12g

Bell Pepper and Egg in a Hole

Prep Time: 5 Minutes | **Cook Time:** 10 Minutes |
Serves: 2

INGREDIENTS:

- ❖ 1 large bell pepper, cut into 1/2-inch rings
- ❖ 4 large eggs
- ❖ Salt and pepper to taste
- ❖ 1 tablespoon olive oil or butter

INSTRUCTIONS:

1. Heat olive oil or butter in a large non-stick skillet over medium heat.
2. Place the bell pepper rings in the skillet and let them sauté for about 1 minute.
3. Crack an egg into the center of each bell pepper ring. Season with salt and pepper.
4. Cover the skillet and cook for 5-7 minutes, or until the egg whites are set but the yolks are still runny (cook longer if you prefer the yolks to be fully set).
5. Carefully remove with a spatula and serve immediately.

NUTRITIONAL INFORMATION (PER SERVING):

Calories: 180 | Carbs: 3g | Fiber: 1g | Net Carbs: 2g
Protein: 11g | Fats: 14g

Bacon and Egg Stuffed Avocado

Prep Time: 15 Minutes | **Cook Time:** 5 Minutes |
Serves: 2

INGREDIENTS:

- ❖ 1 large avocado, halved and pit removed
- ❖ 2 slices of bacon, cooked and crumbled
- ❖ 2 large eggs
- ❖ Salt and pepper to taste
- ❖ Chopped chives or parsley for garnish (optional)

INSTRUCTIONS:

1. Preheat your oven to 425°F (220°C). Scoop out a little flesh from each avocado half to make enough room for the egg.
2. Place the avocado halves in a small baking dish to prevent them from tipping over.
3. Carefully crack an egg into each avocado half. Season with salt and pepper.
4. Bake in the preheated oven for 12-15 minutes, or until the egg whites are set but the yolks are still slightly runny.
5. Sprinkle with crumbled bacon and garnish with chives or parsley before serving.

NUTRITIONAL INFORMATION (PER SERVING):

Calories: 290 | Carbs: 9g | Fiber: 7g | Net Carbs: 2g
Protein: 14g | Fats: 24g

Sautéed Greens with Garlic and Poached Eggs

Prep Time: 10 Minutes | **Cook Time:** 15 Minutes |
Serves: 2

INGREDIENTS:

- ❖ 4 cups mixed greens (kale, spinach, Swiss chard), chopped
- ❖ 2 large eggs
- ❖ 2 cloves garlic, minced
- ❖ 2 tablespoons olive oil
- ❖ Salt and pepper to taste
- ❖ 1 tablespoon white vinegar (for poaching eggs)

INSTRUCTIONS:

1. Heat 1 tablespoon of olive oil in a large skillet over medium heat. Add minced garlic and sauté until fragrant, about 1 minute.
2. Add the mixed greens to the skillet, season with salt and pepper, and sauté until wilted, about 3-5 minutes. Remove from heat and divide the greens between two plates.
3. In a medium saucepan, bring water to a gentle simmer and add the white vinegar. Crack an egg into a small bowl and gently slide it into the simmering water. Repeat with the second egg. Poach the eggs for 3-4 minutes, or until the whites are set but the yolks are still runny.
4. Using a slotted spoon, remove the poached eggs from the water and place one on top of each serving of greens.

5. Drizzle the remaining olive oil over each plate and season with additional salt and pepper if desired. Serve immediately.

Calories: 220 | Carbs: 5g | Fiber: 2g | Net Carbs: 3g
Protein: 12g | Fats: 18g

Broccoli Cheese Breakfast Casserole

Prep Time: 10 Minutes | **Cook Time:** 35 Minutes |
Serves: 6

INGREDIENTS:

- 2 cups broccoli florets, chopped
- 1 cup cheddar cheese, shredded
- 6 large eggs
- 1/2 cup heavy cream
- 1/2 cup almond milk
- Salt and pepper to taste
- 1/4 tsp garlic powder
- 1/4 tsp paprika

INSTRUCTIONS:

1. Preheat your oven to 375°F (190°C). Lightly grease a 9-inch baking dish.
2. Steam the broccoli until just tender, then spread evenly in the bottom of the prepared baking dish. Sprinkle the shredded cheese over the broccoli.
3. In a mixing bowl, whisk together eggs, heavy cream, almond milk, salt, pepper, garlic powder, and paprika. Pour this mixture over the broccoli and cheese.
4. Bake for 35 minutes, or until the center is set and the top is lightly golden. Let it cool for a few minutes before slicing and serving.

NUTRITIONAL INFORMATION (PER SERVING):

Calories: 220 | Carbs: 4g | Fiber: 1g | Net Carbs: 3g
Protein: 14g | Fats: 7g

Whole-Grain Strawberry Pancakes

Prep Time: 15 Minutes | **Cook Time:** 15 Minutes |
Serves: 4

INGREDIENTS:

- 1 cup whole grain flour (choose a low-carb, diabetic-friendly option like almond or coconut flour)
- 2 large eggs
- 1/2 cup unsweetened almond milk
- 1 tsp baking powder
- 1 cup strawberries, diced
- 1/2 tsp vanilla extract
- 2 tbsp erythritol or sweetener of choice
- Butter or oil for cooking

INSTRUCTIONS:

1. In a large bowl, combine the flour, baking powder, and sweetener.
2. In another bowl, whisk together eggs, almond milk, and vanilla extract. Add the wet ingredients to the dry ingredients and stir until just combined. Fold in the diced strawberries.
3. Heat a non-stick skillet over medium heat and grease lightly with butter or oil. Pour 1/4 cup of batter for each pancake, cooking until bubbles form on the surface, then flip and cook until golden brown on the other side.
4. Serve warm with additional strawberries on top if desired.

NUTRITIONAL INFORMATION (PER SERVING):

Calories: 250 | Carbs: 10g | Fiber: 6g | Net Carbs: 4g
Protein: 11g | Fats: 20g

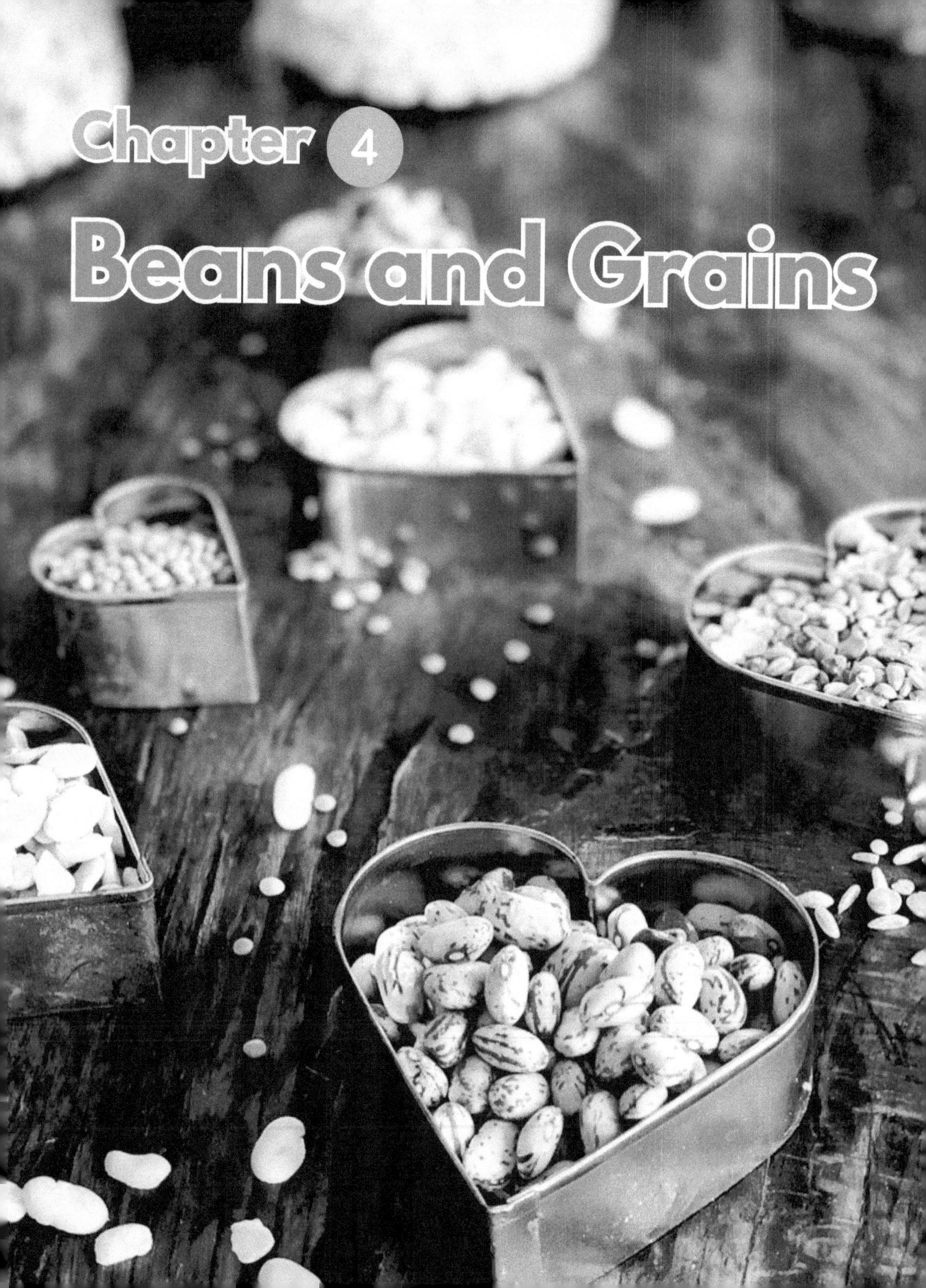

Chapter 4
Beans and Grains

Prep Time: 10 Minutes | **Cook Time:** 15 Minutes | **Serves:** 4

INGREDIENTS:

- 1 large head cauliflower, riced
- 1/4 cup onion, finely diced
- 1/4 cup carrots, finely diced
- 1/4 cup celery, finely diced
- 1/2 cup chicken or vegetable broth
- 2 cloves garlic, minced
- 2 tbsp olive oil
- 1 tsp turmeric (optional for color and flavor)
- Salt and pepper to taste
- Fresh herbs for garnish (parsley, cilantro)

INSTRUCTIONS:

1. Heat olive oil in a large skillet over medium heat. Add onion, carrots, celery, and garlic, sautéing until softened.
2. Stir in the riced cauliflower, turmeric (if using), salt, and pepper. Cook for about 5 minutes, stirring occasionally.
3. Add the broth, cover, and let simmer for about 5-10 minutes or until the cauliflower is tender and the liquid is absorbed.
4. Garnish with fresh herbs before serving.

NUTRITIONAL INFORMATION (PER SERVING):

Calories: 120 | Carbs: 10g | Fiber: 4g | Net Carbs: 6g
Protein: 3g | Fats: 7g

Black Soybean Hummus

Prep Time: 10 Minutes | **Cook Time:** 0 Minute | **Serves:** 8

INGREDIENTS:

- 1 can (15 oz) black soybeans, drained and rinsed
- 2 tablespoons tahini
- 2 tablespoons olive oil
- 1 clove garlic, minced
- Juice of 1 lemon
- 1/2 teaspoon ground cumin
- Salt and pepper to taste
- Water, as needed for consistency

INSTRUCTIONS:

1. Combine black soybeans, tahini, olive oil, minced garlic, lemon juice, and ground cumin in a food processor.
2. Blend until smooth, adding water a tablespoon at a time until desired consistency is reached.
3. Season with salt and pepper to taste.
4. Serve with low-carb vegetables or keto-friendly crackers.

NUTRITIONAL INFORMATION (PER SERVING):

Calories: 100 | Carbs: 5g | Fiber: 3g | Net Carbs: 2g
Protein: 6g | Fats: 7g

Edamame and Quinoa Salad

Prep Time: 15 Minutes | **Cook Time:** 20 Minutes | **Serves:** 4

INGREDIENTS:

- 1 cup quinoa, rinsed
- 2 cups water
- 1 cup edamame, shelled and cooked
- 1 red bell pepper, diced
- 1/4 cup red onion, finely chopped
- 1/4 cup cilantro, chopped
- 2 tablespoons olive oil
- Juice of 1 lime
- Salt and pepper to taste

INSTRUCTIONS:

1. In a saucepan, bring quinoa and water to a boil. Reduce heat, cover, and simmer for 15 minutes or until water is absorbed. Let it cool.
2. In a large bowl, combine cooled quinoa, edamame, red bell pepper, red onion, and cilantro.
3. In a small bowl, whisk together olive oil, lime juice, salt, and pepper. Pour over the salad and toss to coat.
4. Chill in the refrigerator before serving.

Calories: 250 | Carbs: 30g | Fiber: 5g | Net Carbs: 25g
Protein: 10g | Fats: 10g

Chia and Flaxseed Oatmeal

Prep Time: 5 Minutes | **Cook Time:** 5 Minutes | **Serves:** 2

INGREDIENTS:

- 1/4 cup chia seeds
- 1/4 cup ground flaxseeds
- 1 cup unsweetened almond milk
- 1/2 teaspoon cinnamon
- 1 tablespoon erythritol or sweetener of choice
- 1/2 teaspoon vanilla extract
- Fresh berries for topping (optional)

INSTRUCTIONS:

1. In a small saucepan, combine chia seeds, ground flaxseeds, almond milk, cinnamon, and sweetener.
2. Cook over medium heat, stirring constantly until the mixture thickens, about 5 minutes.
3. Remove from heat and stir in vanilla extract.
4. Divide into bowls and top with fresh berries if desired. Serve warm.

NUTRITIONAL INFORMATION (PER SERVING):

Calories: 200 | Carbs: 10g | Fiber: 8g | Net Carbs: 2g
Protein: 6g | Fats: 14g

Low-Carb Refried Beans

Prep Time: 10 Minutes | **Cook Time:** 15 Minutes | **Serves:** 6

INGREDIENTS:

- 2 cans (15 oz each) black soybeans, drained and rinsed
- 2 tablespoons olive oil
- 1/2 onion, finely chopped
- 2 cloves garlic, minced
- 1 teaspoon ground cumin
- 1/2 teaspoon chili powder
- Salt and pepper to taste
- 1/4 cup water or vegetable broth

INSTRUCTIONS:

1. Heat olive oil in a skillet over medium heat. Add onions and garlic, sautéing until softened, about 5 minutes.
2. Add the black soybeans, cumin, chili powder, salt, and pepper. Cook for another 5 minutes, stirring occasionally.
3. Add water or vegetable broth, then use a potato masher or the back of a spoon to mash the beans to your desired consistency. Cook for an additional 5 minutes, adjusting seasoning if needed.
4. Serve warm as a side dish or use as a filling for low-carb tacos or burritos.

NUTRITIONAL INFORMATION (PER SERVING):

Calories: 150 | Carbs: 8g | Fiber: 5g | Net Carbs: 3g
Protein: 11g | Fats: 9g

Spicy Roasted Chickpeas

Prep Time: 5 Minutes | **Cook Time:** 40 Minutes | **Serves:** 4

INGREDIENTS:

- 1 can (15 oz) chickpeas, drained, rinsed, and patted dry
- 2 tablespoons olive oil
- 1/2 teaspoon smoked paprika
- 1/2 teaspoon ground cumin
- 1/4 teaspoon cayenne pepper (adjust to taste)
- Salt to taste

INSTRUCTIONS:

1. Preheat oven to 400°F (200°C) and line a baking sheet with parchment paper.
2. In a bowl, toss the chickpeas with olive oil, smoked paprika, cumin, cayenne pepper, and salt until evenly coated.
3. Spread the chickpeas out in a single layer on the prepared baking sheet.
4. Roast in the oven for 30-40 minutes, shaking the pan

or stirring halfway through, until the chickpeas are crispy and golden.

5. Let cool before serving as a crunchy snack or salad topping.

Calories: 180 | Carbs: 20g | Fiber: 5g | Net Carbs: 15g
Protein: 6g | Fats: 8g

Shirataki Rice Pudding

Prep Time: 5 Minutes | **Cook Time:** 15 Minutes | **Serves:** 5

INGREDIENTS:

- 1 package (8 oz) shirataki rice (miracle rice), rinsed and drained
- 1 cup unsweetened almond milk
- 1/4 cup heavy cream
- 1 cinnamon stick or 1/2 teaspoon ground cinnamon
- 1/4 teaspoon vanilla extract
- 2 tablespoons erythritol or sweetener of choice
- Pinch of salt
- Ground cinnamon for garnish (optional)

INSTRUCTIONS:

1. In a saucepan, combine the shirataki rice, almond milk, heavy cream, cinnamon stick, vanilla extract, sweetener, and a pinch of salt.
2. Bring to a simmer over medium heat, stirring occasionally.
3. Reduce the heat to low and continue to cook, stirring frequently, for about 10-15 minutes, or until the mixture thickens to your desired consistency.
4. Remove the cinnamon stick if used and serve the rice pudding warm or chilled, garnished with ground cinnamon if desired.

NUTRITIONAL INFORMATION (PER SERVING):

Calories: 150 | Carbs: 1g | Fiber: 0g | Net Carbs: 1g
Protein: 1g | Fats: 15g

INSTRUCTIONS:

1. Preheat your oven to 375°F (190°C).
2. Heat olive oil in an oven-safe skillet over medium heat. Sauté onions until translucent.
3. Add spinach and cook until wilted.
4. In a bowl, whisk together eggs, heavy cream, salt, and pepper.
5. Pour the egg mixture over the spinach and onions in the skillet. Sprinkle feta cheese on top.
6. Cook without stirring for about 2-3 minutes until the edges start to set.
7. Transfer the skillet to the oven and bake for 15-17 minutes, or until the frittata is set and lightly golden.
8. Let it cool slightly before cutting into wedges and serving.

NUTRITIONAL INFORMATION (PER SERVING):

Calories: 220 | Carbs: 4g | Fiber: 1g | Net Carbs: 3g
Protein: 12g | Fats: 18g

Lentil and Mushroom Stuffed Peppers

Prep Time: 15 Minutes | **Cook Time:** 30 Minutes | **Serves:** 4

INGREDIENTS:

- 4 large bell peppers, tops cut off and seeds removed
- 1 cup cooked lentils (use a low-carb alternative if desired)
- 1 cup mushrooms, finely chopped
- 1 cup spinach, chopped
- 1/2 cup onion, diced
- 2 cloves garlic, minced
- 1/2 cup low-carb tomato sauce
- 1/2 cup shredded mozzarella cheese (optional)
- 2 tablespoons olive oil
- Salt and pepper to taste

INSTRUCTIONS:

1. Preheat your oven to 375°F (190°C).
2. Heat olive oil in a skillet over medium heat. Add onions and garlic, sautéing until translucent.
3. Add mushrooms and cook until they release their moisture and start to brown.
4. Stir in the cooked lentils, spinach, and tomato sauce. Season with salt and pepper. Cook until the spinach is wilted.

5. Place stuffed peppers in a baking dish and bake for 25-30 minutes, or until the peppers are tender and the cheese is melted and bubbly.
6. Serve warm.

Calories: 220 | Carbs: 20g | Fiber: 8g | Net Carbs: 12g
Protein: 10g | Fats: 10g

Broccoli and Cheese Quinoa Bites

Prep Time: 15 Minutes | **Cook Time:** 20 Minutes | **Serves:** 12 Bites

INGREDIENTS:

- 1 cup cooked quinoa (use cauliflower rice for a lower carb option)
- 1 cup broccoli, finely chopped and steamed
- 1/2 cup sharp cheddar cheese, shredded
- 2 large eggs
- 1/4 cup almond flour
- 1/2 teaspoon garlic powder
- Salt and pepper to taste

INSTRUCTIONS:

1. Preheat your oven to 350°F (175°C) and grease a mini muffin tin.
2. In a large bowl, combine the cooked quinoa or cauliflower rice, steamed broccoli, shredded cheese, eggs, almond flour, garlic powder, salt, and pepper.
3. Spoon the mixture into the prepared mini muffin tin, pressing down to compact.
4. Bake for 18-20 minutes, or until the edges are golden and the bites are set.
5. Let cool for a few minutes before removing from the tin. Serve warm.

NUTRITIONAL INFORMATION (PER SERVING):

Calories: 60 | Carbs: 2g | Fiber: 1g | Net Carbs: 1g
Protein: 4g | Fats: 4g

Mung Bean Sprout Salad

Prep Time: 10 Minutes | **Cook Time:** 0 Minute | **Serves:** 4

INGREDIENTS:

- 2 cups mung bean sprouts, rinsed and drained
- 1 cucumber, thinly sliced
- 1 carrot, julienned
- 1/4 cup cilantro, chopped
- 2 tablespoons green onions, chopped

For the dressing:

- 2 tablespoons soy sauce (or tamari for gluten-free)
- 1 tablespoon sesame oil
- 1 tablespoon rice vinegar
- 1 teaspoon erythritol or sweetener of choice
- 1 clove garlic, minced
- 1 teaspoon ginger, grated

INSTRUCTIONS:

1. In a large bowl, combine mung bean sprouts, cucumber slices, julienned carrot, chopped cilantro, and green onions.
2. In a small bowl, whisk together soy sauce, sesame oil, rice vinegar, sweetener, minced garlic, and grated ginger to create the dressing.
3. Pour the dressing over the salad and toss well to coat all the ingredients.
4. Chill in the refrigerator for about 30 minutes before serving to allow the flavors to meld.

NUTRITIONAL INFORMATION (PER SERVING):

Calories: 80 | Carbs: 6g | Fiber: 1g | Net Carbs: 5g
Protein: 3g | Fats: 5g

Almond and Coconut Porridge

Prep Time: 5 Minutes | **Cook Time:** 10 Minutes | **Serves:** 2

- 1/2 cup almond flour
- 1/4 cup shredded coconut, unsweetened
- 1 cup unsweetened almond milk
- 1/4 cup coconut cream
- Pinch of salt
- 1 tablespoon erythritol or sweetener of choice
- 1/2 teaspoon vanilla extract
- Cinnamon for garnish (optional)
- Fresh berries for topping (optional)

INSTRUCTIONS:

1. In a saucepan, combine almond flour, shredded coconut, almond milk, coconut cream, sweetener, vanilla extract, and a pinch of salt.
2. Cook over medium heat, stirring constantly to prevent lumps, until the mixture thickens to a porridge-like consistency, about 5-10 minutes.
3. Serve warm, garnished with a sprinkle of cinnamon and topped with fresh berries if desired.

NUTRITIONAL INFORMATION (PER SERVING):

Calories: 300 | Carbs: 10g | Fiber: 4g | Net Carbs: 6g
Protein: 6g | Fats: 28g

Hemp Seed Tabouleh

Prep Time: 15 Minutes | **Cook Time:** 0 Minute |
Serves: 4

INGREDIENTS:

- 1 cup hemp seeds
- 2 cups parsley, finely chopped
- 1/2 cup mint leaves, finely chopped
- 1/4 cup onion, finely diced
- 2 tomatoes, diced
- 2 tablespoons olive oil
- Juice of 1 lemon
- Salt and pepper to taste

INSTRUCTIONS:

1. In a large bowl, combine hemp seeds, chopped parsley, mint, diced onion, and tomatoes.

2. Drizzle with olive oil and lemon juice, then season with salt and pepper.
3. Toss everything together until well mixed. Adjust seasoning if necessary.
4. Serve immediately or let it sit for a while to allow flavors to meld.

NUTRITIONAL INFORMATION (PER SERVING):

Calories: 250 | Carbs: 8g | Fiber: 4g | Net Carbs: 4g
Protein: 15g | Fats: 20g

Black Bean and Avocado Lettuce Wrap

Prep Time: 10 Minutes | **Cook Time:** 0 Minutes |
Serves: 4

INGREDIENTS:

- 1 can (15 oz) black beans, rinsed and drained
- 1/2 cup corn kernels (optional, omit for lower carbs)
- 1/4 cup red onion, finely chopped
- 1 ripe avocado, diced
- 1/4 cup cilantro, chopped
- 1 lime, juiced
- Salt and pepper to taste
- 8 large lettuce leaves (romaine or iceberg)

INSTRUCTIONS:

1. In a bowl, gently mix together black beans, diced avocado, corn (if using), red onion, cilantro, and lime juice. Season with salt and pepper to taste.
2. Carefully spoon the mixture into the center of each lettuce leaf, folding in the sides to create a wrap.
3. Serve immediately, with additional lime wedges on the side if desired.

NUTRITIONAL INFORMATION (PER SERVING):

Calories: 150 | Carbs: 18g | Fiber: 8g | Net Carbs: 10g
Protein: 6g | Fats: 7g

Spaghetti Squash and Lentil Bolognese

Prep Time: 15 Minutes | **Cook Time:** 45 Minutes | **Serves:** 4

INGREDIENTS:

- 1 large spaghetti squash
- 1 cup dried green or brown lentils, rinsed
- 2 tablespoons olive oil
- 1 onion, diced
- 2 cloves garlic, minced
- 1 carrot, diced
- 1 celery stalk, diced
- 1 can (28 oz) crushed tomatoes
- 1 teaspoon dried oregano
- 1 teaspoon dried basil
- Salt and pepper to taste
- Fresh parsley for garnish

INSTRUCTIONS:

1. Preheat your oven to 400°F (200°C). Halve the spaghetti squash lengthwise and scoop out the seeds. Place the halves cut-side down on a baking sheet and roast until tender, about 30-40 minutes.
2. Meanwhile, cook the lentils in boiling water until tender, about 20 minutes. Drain and set aside.
3. Heat olive oil in a large skillet over medium heat. Add onion, garlic, carrot, and celery. Cook until softened, about 5 minutes.
4. Add the crushed tomatoes, oregano, basil, cooked lentils, salt, and pepper to the skillet. Simmer for 10-15 minutes, allowing flavors to meld.
5. Once the spaghetti squash is cool enough to handle, use a fork to scrape the insides into strands.
6. Serve the lentil Bolognese sauce over the spaghetti squash strands. Garnish with fresh parsley.

NUTRITIONAL INFORMATION (PER SERVING):

Calories: 280 | Carbs: 45g | Fiber: 12g | Net Carbs: 33g
Protein: 14g | Fats: 7g

Thai Red Lentils

Prep Time: 10 Minutes | **Cook Time:** 25 Minutes | **Serves:** 4

INGREDIENTS:

- 1 cup red lentils, rinsed
- 1 tablespoon coconut oil
- 1 onion, diced
- 2 cloves garlic, minced
- 1 tablespoon Thai red curry paste
- 1 can (14 oz) coconut milk
- 2 cups vegetable broth
- Juice of 1 lime
- Salt to taste
- Fresh cilantro for garnish

INSTRUCTIONS:

1. Heat coconut oil in a pot over medium heat. Add onion and garlic, cooking until soft.
2. Stir in the red curry paste and cook for 1 minute.
3. Add red lentils, coconut milk, and vegetable broth. Bring to a boil, then reduce heat and simmer until lentils are tender, about 20 minutes.
4. Stir in lime juice and season with salt to taste.
5. Serve garnished with fresh cilantro.

NUTRITIONAL INFORMATION (PER SERVING):

Calories: 350 | Carbs: 35g | Fiber: 15g | Net Carbs: 20g
Protein: 15g | Fats: 18g

Eggplant and Chickpea Curry

Prep Time: 15 Minutes | **Cook Time:** 30 Minutes | **Serves:** 4

INGREDIENTS:

- 1 large eggplant, cubed
- 1 can (15 oz) chickpeas, drained and rinsed
- 2 tablespoons olive oil
- 1 tablespoon curry powder
- 2 cloves garlic, minced
- 1 tablespoon ginger, grated
- 1 onion, diced
- 1 can (14 oz) diced tomatoes
- 1 can (14 oz) coconut milk
- Salt and pepper to taste
- Fresh cilantro for garnish

INSTRUCTIONS:

1. Heat olive oil in a large skillet over medium heat. Add

onion, garlic, and ginger, cooking until softened.

2. Stir in curry powder and cook for 1 minute.
3. Add eggplant and cook for 5 minutes, stirring occasionally.
4. Stir in chickpeas, diced tomatoes, and coconut milk. Season with salt and pepper.
5. Bring to a simmer and cook until the eggplant is tender and the sauce has thickened, about 20 minutes.
6. Serve garnished with fresh cilantro.

NUTRITIONAL INFORMATION (PER SERVING):

Calories: 330 | Carbs: 30g | Fiber: 10g | Net Carbs: 20g
Protein: 9g | Fats: 20g

Zucchini and Black Bean Veggie Burgers

Prep Time: 20 Minutes | **Cook Time:** 10 Minutes |
Serves: 4

INGREDIENTS:

- ❖ 1 cup black beans, drained and rinsed
- ❖ 1 medium zucchini, grated and excess moisture squeezed out
- ❖ 1/2 cup almond flour
- ❖ 1 egg, beaten
- ❖ 2 green onions, finely chopped
- ❖ 1 clove garlic, minced
- ❖ 1 tsp cumin
- ❖ Salt and pepper to taste
- ❖ 1 tbsp olive oil for cooking

INSTRUCTIONS:

1. Mash the black beans in a bowl until mostly smooth.
2. Stir in the grated zucchini, almond flour, beaten egg, green onions, garlic, cumin, salt, and pepper until well combined.
3. Form the mixture into 4 patties.
4. Heat olive oil in a skillet over medium heat. Cook the patties for about 5 minutes on each side, or until they are golden brown and heated through.
5. Serve the veggie burgers on low-carb buns or wrapped in lettuce leaves with your favorite toppings.

NUTRITIONAL INFORMATION (PER SERVING):

Calories: 220 | Carbs: 15g | Fiber: 7g | Net Carbs: 8g
Protein: 10g | Fats: 14g

Cauliflower and Cheese Bake

Prep Time: 15 Minutes | **Cook Time:** 25 Minutes |
Serves: 6

INGREDIENTS:

- ❖ 1 large head cauliflower, cut into florets
- ❖ 1 cup heavy cream
- ❖ 1 cup shredded sharp cheddar cheese
- ❖ 2 cloves garlic, minced
- ❖ 1/2 cup grated Parmesan cheese
- ❖ Salt and pepper to taste
- ❖ 1/2 tsp paprika (optional for garnish)

INSTRUCTIONS:

1. Preheat your oven to 375°F (190°C). Lightly grease a baking dish.
2. Steam the cauliflower florets until just tender, about 5-7 minutes. Then, transfer them to the baking dish.
3. In a saucepan, combine heavy cream, cheddar cheese, Parmesan cheese, and minced garlic. Cook over low heat, stirring until the cheese melts and the mixture is smooth.
4. Pour the cheese sauce over the cauliflower in the baking dish. Season with salt and pepper.
5. Sprinkle paprika on top for color, if desired.
6. Bake for 20-25 minutes, or until the top is golden and bubbly.
7. Serve hot as a side dish.

NUTRITIONAL INFORMATION (PER SERVING):

Calories: 300 | Carbs: 8g | Fiber: 3g | Net Carbs: 5g
Protein: 12g | Fats: 25g

Mushroom Hazelnut Rice

Prep Time: 10 Minutes | **Cook Time:** 20 Minutes |
Serves: 4

INGREDIENTS:

- ❖ 1 cup cauliflower rice (as a low-carb substitute for regular rice)
- ❖ 1/2 onion, diced
- ❖ 1 cup mushrooms, sliced
- ❖ 1/4 cup hazelnuts, chopped

* 2 tbsp olive oil
* Fresh parsley for garnish
* 1 clove garlic, minced
* Salt and pepper to taste

1. Heat olive oil in a large skillet over medium heat. Add the diced onion and minced garlic, sautéing until translucent.
2. Add the sliced mushrooms to the skillet and cook until they release their moisture and begin to brown.
3. Stir in the cauliflower rice and chopped hazelnuts, cooking for an additional 5-7 minutes, or until the cauliflower rice is tender.
4. Season with salt and pepper to taste.
5. Garnish with fresh parsley before serving.

NUTRITIONAL INFORMATION (PER SERVING):

Calories: 180 | Carbs: 8g | Fiber: 3g | Net Carbs: 5g
Protein: 4g | Fats: 15g

Green Bean Almondine

Prep Time: 10 Minutes | **Cook Time:** 10 Minutes | **Serves:** 4

INGREDIENTS:

* 1 lb green beans, trimmed
* 1/4 cup sliced almonds
* 2 tablespoons butter
* 1 clove garlic, minced
* Salt and pepper to taste
* Lemon zest for garnish (optional)

INSTRUCTIONS:

1. Blanch the green beans in boiling water for 2-3 minutes until bright green and tender-crisp. Drain and plunge into ice water to stop the cooking process. Drain again and set aside.
2. In a skillet, melt the butter over medium heat. Add the garlic and sliced almonds, sautéing until the almonds are golden brown.
3. Add the blanched green beans to the skillet, tossing to coat with the butter, garlic, and almonds. Season with salt and pepper to taste.
4. Cook for an additional 2-3 minutes, until the green beans are heated through.
5. Garnish with lemon zest if desired before serving.

NUTRITIONAL INFORMATION (PER SERVING):

Calories: 120 | Carbs: 8g | Fiber: 3g | Net Carbs: 5g
Protein: 6g | Fats: 9g

Stuffed Bell Peppers with Quinoa and Spinach

Prep Time: 15 Minutes | **Cook Time:** 30 Minutes | **Serves:** 4

INGREDIENTS:

* 4 bell peppers, tops removed and seeded
* 1 cup cooked quinoa (use cauliflower rice for a lower carb option)
* 1 cup spinach, chopped
* 1 clove garlic, minced
* 1/2 cup onion, diced
* 1/2 cup feta cheese, crumbled
* 1/4 cup pine nuts or chopped walnuts (optional)
* 1 tablespoon olive oil
* Salt and pepper to taste

INSTRUCTIONS:

1. Preheat your oven to 375°F (190°C).
2. In a skillet, heat the olive oil over medium heat. Add the onion and garlic, sautéing until softened.
3. Stir in the spinach and cook until wilted. Remove from heat and let it cool slightly.
4. In a bowl, combine the cooked quinoa (or cauliflower rice), spinach mixture, feta cheese, and nuts if using. Season with salt and pepper.
5. Stuff the mixture into the hollowed-out bell peppers and place them in a baking dish.
6. Bake for 25-30 minutes, or until the peppers are tender and the filling is heated through.
7. Serve warm.

NUTRITIONAL INFORMATION (PER SERVING):

Calories: 180 | Carbs: 12g | Fiber: 3g | Net Carbs: 9g
Protein: 6g | Fats: 12g

Kale and White Bean Soup

Prep Time: 10 Minutes | **Cook Time:** 30 Minutes | **Serves:** 6

- ❖ 1 tablespoon olive oil
- ❖ 1 onion, diced
- ❖ 2 carrots, diced
- ❖ 2 stalks celery, diced
- ❖ 2 cloves garlic, minced
- ❖ 1 can (15 oz) white beans, drained and rinsed
- ❖ 4 cups vegetable broth
- ❖ 4 cups kale, chopped
- ❖ 1 teaspoon dried thyme
- ❖ Salt and pepper to taste
- ❖ Parmesan cheese for garnish (optional)

INSTRUCTIONS:

1. Heat the olive oil in a large pot over medium heat. Add the onion, carrots, and celery, cooking until softened, about 5 minutes.
2. Add the garlic and cook for an additional minute until fragrant.
3. Stir in the white beans, vegetable broth, and thyme. Bring to a simmer.
4. Add the chopped kale to the pot and cook until wilted, about 5-10 minutes.
5. Season the soup with salt and pepper to taste.
6. Serve hot, garnished with grated Parmesan cheese if desired.

NUTRITIONAL INFORMATION (PER SERVING):

Calories: 150 | Carbs: 24g | Fiber: 6g | Net Carbs: 18g
Protein: 8g | Fats: 3g

Roasted Brussels Sprouts with Pecans

Prep Time: 10 Minutes | **Cook Time:** 20 Minutes |
Serves: 4

INGREDIENTS:

- ❖ 1 lb Brussels sprouts, trimmed and halved
- ❖ 1/2 cup pecans, roughly chopped
- ❖ 2 tablespoons olive oil
- ❖ Salt and pepper to taste
- ❖ Balsamic vinegar for drizzling (optional)

INSTRUCTIONS:

1. Preheat your oven to 400°F (200°C).
2. In a large bowl, toss the Brussels sprouts and pecans with olive oil, salt, and pepper until well coated.
3. Spread the mixture in a single layer on a baking sheet.
4. Roast in the preheated oven for 20 minutes, or until the Brussels sprouts are tender and the edges are crispy. Stir halfway through to ensure even roasting.
5. Drizzle with balsamic vinegar if desired before serving.

NUTRITIONAL INFORMATION (PER SERVING):

Calories: 180 | Carbs: 10g | Fiber: 4g | Net Carbs: 6g
Protein: 4g | Fats: 15g

Green Chickpea Falafel

Prep Time: 20 Minutes | **Cook Time:** 10 Minutes |
Serves: 4

INGREDIENTS:

- ❖ 2 cups green chickpeas (fresh or if using dried, soaked overnight and drained)
- ❖ 1 onion, chopped
- ❖ 2 cloves garlic, minced
- ❖ 1/4 cup fresh parsley, chopped
- ❖ 1/4 cup fresh cilantro, chopped
- ❖ 1 teaspoon ground cumin
- ❖ 1 teaspoon ground coriander
- ❖ Salt and pepper to taste
- ❖ Olive oil for frying

INSTRUCTIONS:

1. In a food processor, combine the green chickpeas, onion, garlic, parsley, cilantro, cumin, coriander, salt, and pepper. Pulse until the mixture is finely ground but not pureed.
2. Form the mixture into small balls or patties.
3. Heat a thin layer of olive oil in a skillet over medium heat. Fry the falafel in batches, turning once, until golden and crispy, about 5 minutes.
4. Drain on paper towels and serve hot.

NUTRITIONAL INFORMATION (PER SERVING):

Calories: 250 | Carbs: 20g | Fiber: 8g | Net Carbs: 32g
Protein: 10g | Fats: 10g

Moroccan-Spiced Cauliflower and Almond Couscous

Prep Time: 15 Minutes | **Cook Time:** 10 Minutes | **Serves:** 4

INGREDIENTS:

- 1 large head cauliflower, riced
- 1/2 cup almonds, chopped and toasted
- 1/4 cup raisins (optional, omit for lower carbs)
- 1/4 cup fresh parsley, chopped
- 1 teaspoon ground cumin
- 1/2 teaspoon ground cinnamon
- 1/2 teaspoon ground turmeric
- 2 tablespoons olive oil
- Salt and pepper to taste

INSTRUCTIONS:

1. Heat olive oil in a large skillet over medium heat. Add the riced cauliflower, cumin, cinnamon, and turmeric. Cook, stirring occasionally, for 5-7 minutes or until the cauliflower is tender.
2. Stir in the toasted almonds, raisins (if using), and chopped parsley. Season with salt and pepper to taste.
3. Cook for an additional 2-3 minutes, allowing the flavors to meld.
4. Serve warm as a side dish, garnished with extra parsley if desired.

NUTRITIONAL INFORMATION (PER SERVING):

Calories: 180 | Carbs: 12g | Fiber: 5g | Net Carbs: 7g
Protein: 6g | Fats: 14g

Veggies and Kasha with Balsamic Vinaigrette

Prep Time: 15 Minutes | **Cook Time:** 20 Minutes | **Serves:** 4

INGREDIENTS:

- 2 cups vegetable broth
- 1 red bell pepper, diced
- 1 zucchini, diced
- 1 yellow squash, diced
- 1 cup kasha (buckwheat groats; for a lower-carb option, consider using cauliflower rice)
- 2 tablespoons olive oil
- 1 garlic clove, minced
- 1/4 cup red onion, finely chopped
- 2 tablespoons olive oil
- 3 tablespoons balsamic vinegar
- Salt and pepper to taste
- Fresh parsley, chopped for garnish

INSTRUCTIONS:

1. In a saucepan, bring vegetable broth to a boil. Add kasha and simmer, covered on low heat for about 10-15 minutes, or until the liquid is absorbed. Fluff with a fork and set aside to cool.
2. In a skillet, heat 1 tablespoon olive oil over medium heat. Sauté red bell pepper, zucchini, and yellow squash until tender, about 5-7 minutes. Season with salt and pepper.
3. In a small bowl, whisk together 1 tablespoon olive oil, balsamic vinegar, minced garlic, salt, and pepper to make the vinaigrette.
4. In a large bowl, combine cooked kasha, sautéed vegetables, and red onion. Pour the balsamic vinaigrette over the mixture and toss to coat evenly.
5. Garnish with fresh parsley before serving.

NUTRITIONAL INFORMATION (PER SERVING):

Calories: 150 | Carbs: 10g | Fiber: 3g | Net Carbs: 7g
Protein: 3g | Fats: 11g

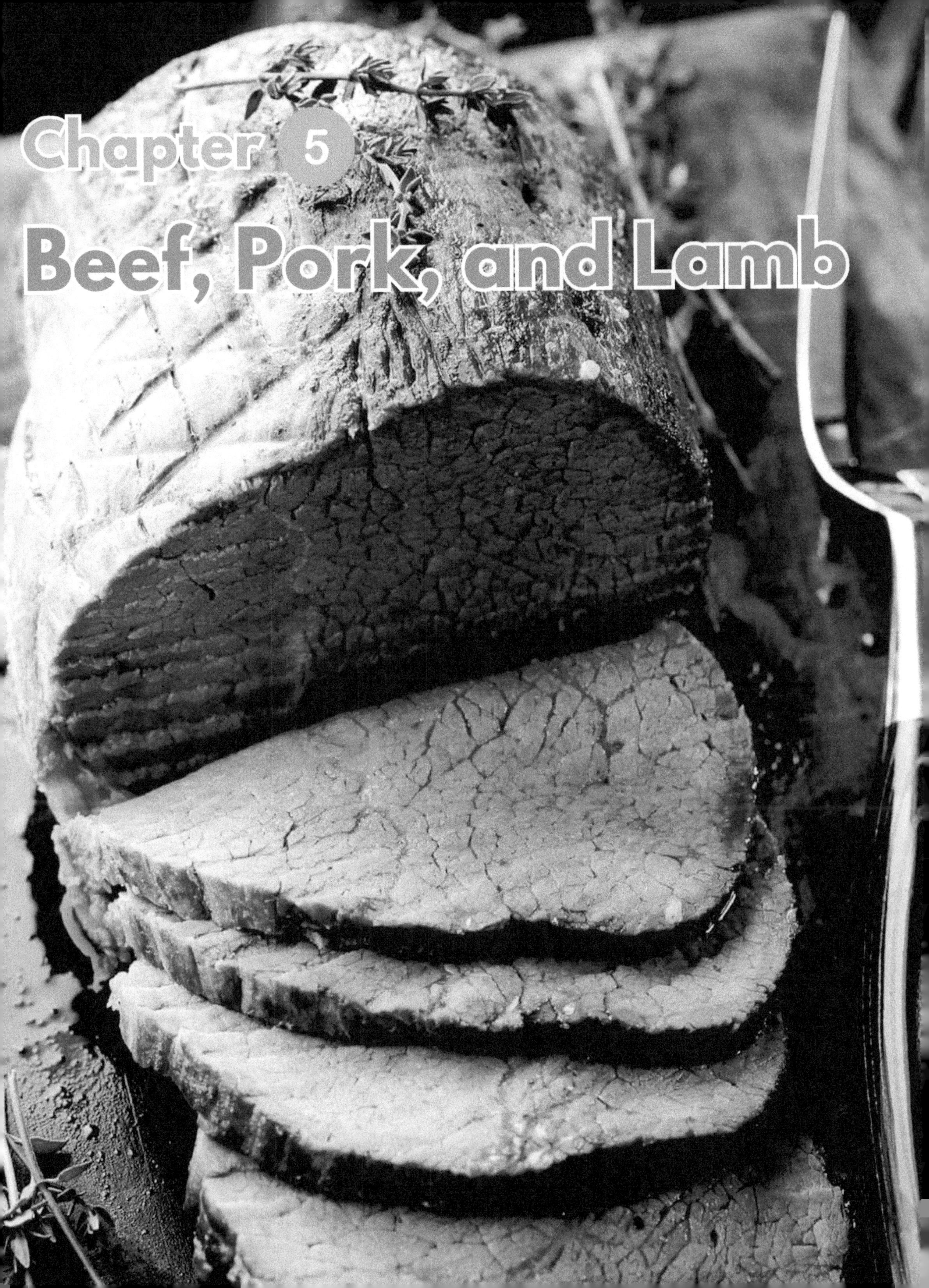
Chapter 5
Beef, Pork, and Lamb

Beef Stir-Fry with Broccoli and Mushrooms

Prep Time: 15 Minutes | **Cook Time:** 10 Minutes | **Serves:** 4

INGREDIENTS:

- 1 lb beef sirloin, thinly sliced
- 2 cups broccoli florets
- 1 cup mushrooms, sliced
- 1 bell pepper, sliced
- 2 tablespoons soy sauce (or tamari for gluten-free)
- 2 cloves garlic, minced
- 1 tablespoon sesame oil
- 1 teaspoon ginger, grated
- Salt and pepper to taste
- 1 tablespoon olive oil for cooking

INSTRUCTIONS:

1. Heat olive oil in a large skillet or wok over high heat. Add the beef slices and stir-fry until browned, about 3-4 minutes. Remove beef and set aside.
2. In the same skillet, add a bit more oil if needed and stir-fry the broccoli, mushrooms, and bell pepper until they start to soften, about 3-5 minutes.
3. Add the garlic and ginger, cooking for another minute until fragrant.
4. Return the beef to the skillet. Add soy sauce and sesame oil, stirring to combine all the ingredients. Cook for another 2-3 minutes.
5. Season with salt and pepper to taste. Serve hot.

NUTRITIONAL INFORMATION (PER SERVING):

Calories: 250 | Carbs: 6g | Fiber: 2g | Net Carbs: 4g Protein: 25g | Fats: 14g

Pork Tenderloin with Brussels Sprouts

Prep Time: 10 Minutes | **Cook Time:** 25 Minutes | **Serves:** 4

INGREDIENTS:

- 1 pork tenderloin (about 1 lb)
- 2 cups Brussels sprouts, halved
- 2 tablespoons olive oil, divided
- 2 cloves garlic, minced
- Salt and pepper to taste
- 1 teaspoon thyme

INSTRUCTIONS:

1. Preheat your oven to 400°F (200°C).
2. Season the pork tenderloin with salt, pepper, and thyme.
3. Heat 1 tablespoon olive oil in a skillet over medium-high heat. Sear the tenderloin on all sides until golden brown, about 5-7 minutes.
4. In a separate bowl, toss the Brussels sprouts with the remaining olive oil, garlic, salt, and pepper.
5. Place the seared tenderloin in a baking dish, surrounded by the seasoned Brussels sprouts.
6. Roast in the preheated oven for about 18-20 minutes, or until the pork reaches an internal temperature of 145°F (63°C).
7. Let the pork rest for a few minutes before slicing. Serve with the roasted Brussels sprouts.

NUTRITIONAL INFORMATION (PER SERVING):

Calories: 240 | Carbs: 6g | Fiber: 2g | Net Carbs: 4g Protein: 30g | Fats: 11g

Lamb Chops with Rosemary and Garlic

Prep Time: 10 Minutes | **Cook Time:** 10 Minutes | **Serves:** 4

INGREDIENTS:

- 8 lamb chops
- 2 tablespoons olive oil
- 2 tablespoons fresh rosemary, chopped
- 2 cloves garlic, minced
- Salt and pepper to taste
- Lemon wedges for serving

INSTRUCTIONS:

1. In a small bowl, mix together olive oil, minced garlic, chopped rosemary, salt, and pepper. Rub this mixture over the lamb chops and let them marinate for at least 30 minutes, or up to a few hours in the refrigerator.
2. Heat a grill pan or skillet over medium-high heat. Grill the lamb chops for 3-5 minutes on each side for medium-rare, or until they reach your desired level of

3. Let the lamb chops rest for a few minutes before serving.
4. Serve with lemon wedges on the side.

Calories: 310 | Carbs: 1g | Fiber: 0g | Net Carbs: 1g
Protein: 25g | Fats: 23g

Stuffed Bell Peppers with Ground Beef

Prep Time: 15 Minutes | **Cook Time:** 35 Minutes | **Serves:** 4

INGREDIENTS:

- 4 large bell peppers, tops removed and seeded
- 1 lb ground beef
- 1/2 cup onion, finely chopped
- 2 cloves garlic, minced
- 1 cup cauliflower rice
- 1 can (14 oz) diced tomatoes, drained
- 1 teaspoon cumin
- 1 teaspoon paprika
- Salt and pepper to taste
- 1/2 cup shredded cheese (optional)

INSTRUCTIONS:

1. Preheat your oven to 375°F (190°C).
2. In a skillet over medium heat, cook ground beef, onion, and garlic until the beef is browned and the onion is soft.
3. Stir in the cauliflower rice, diced tomatoes, cumin, paprika, salt, and pepper. Cook for an additional 5 minutes.
4. Stuff the mixture into the hollowed-out bell peppers. Place the peppers in a baking dish.
5. Bake for 25-30 minutes, until the peppers are tender. If using cheese, sprinkle it on top during the last 5 minutes of baking.
6. Serve hot.

NUTRITIONAL INFORMATION (PER SERVING):

Calories: 280 | Carbs: 12g | Fiber: 3g | Net Carbs: 9g
Protein: 25g | Fats: 16g

Easy Beef Curry

Prep Time: 10 Minutes | **Cook Time:** 60 Minutes | **Serves:** 4

INGREDIENTS:

- 1 lb beef stew meat, cubed
- 1 tablespoon coconut oil
- 1 onion, chopped
- 2 cloves garlic, minced
- 2 tablespoons curry powder
- 1 can (14 oz) coconut milk
- 1 cup beef broth
- Salt and pepper to taste
- Fresh cilantro for garnish

INSTRUCTIONS:

1. In a large pot, heat the coconut oil over medium heat. Add the beef and brown on all sides.
2. Add the chopped onion and minced garlic to the pot and cook until softened.
3. Stir in the curry powder, coating the beef and onions.
4. Pour in the coconut milk and beef broth. Bring to a simmer.
5. Reduce the heat, cover, and simmer for about 1 hour, or until the beef is tender.
6. Season with salt and pepper to taste. Garnish with fresh cilantro before serving.
7. Serve over cauliflower rice for a complete low-carb meal.

NUTRITIONAL INFORMATION (PER SERVING):

Calories: 380 | Carbs: 8g | Fiber: 1g | Net Carbs: 7g
Protein: 25g | Fats: 28g

Bacon-Wrapped Asparagus

Prep Time: 10 Minutes | **Cook Time:** 20 Minutes | **Serves:** 4

INGREDIENTS:

- 16 asparagus spears, trimmed
- 8 slices of bacon, halved crosswise
- Salt and pepper to taste
- Olive oil for drizzling

INSTRUCTIONS:

1. Preheat your oven to 400°F (200°C). Line a baking sheet with parchment paper.
2. Wrap each asparagus spear with a half slice of bacon, starting from the bottom of the spear and spiraling up to the tip.
3. Place the bacon-wrapped asparagus on the prepared baking sheet. Lightly drizzle with olive oil and season with salt and pepper.
4. Bake for 20 minutes, or until the bacon is crispy and the asparagus is tender.
5. Serve hot as a side dish or appetizer.

NUTRITIONAL INFORMATION (PER SERVING):

Calories: 160 | Carbs: 2g | Fiber: 1g | Net Carbs: 1g
Protein: 10g | Fats: 12g

Grilled Ribeye with Herb Butter

Prep Time: 15 Minutes | **Cook Time:** 10 Minutes |
Serves: 4

INGREDIENTS:

- 4 ribeye steaks (about 8 oz each)
- 4 tablespoons herb butter
- Salt and pepper to taste

INSTRUCTIONS:

1. Combine softened butter with minced garlic, chopped parsley, thyme, and a squeeze of lemon juice, then chill.
2. Preheat your grill to high heat.
3. Season the ribeye steaks generously with salt and pepper.
4. Place the steaks on the grill and cook for about 4-5 minutes per side for medium-rare, or until they reach your desired level of doneness.
5. Remove the steaks from the grill and let them rest for a few minutes.
6. Top each steak with a tablespoon of herb butter before serving. The butter will melt over the hot steak, adding flavor.

NUTRITIONAL INFORMATION (PER SERVING):

Calories: 500 | Carbs: 0g | Fiber: 0g | Net Carbs: 0g
Protein: 45g | Fats: 35g

Spicy Pork Ribs with Cabbage Slaw

Prep Time: 20 Minutes | **Cook Time:** 30 Minutes |
Serves: 4

INGREDIENTS:

Ingredients for Spicy Pork Ribs:

- 2 lbs pork ribs
- 2 tablespoons olive oil
- 2 tablespoons paprika
- 1 tablespoon cayenne pepper (adjust to taste)
- 1 tablespoon garlic powder
- Salt and pepper to taste

Ingredients for Cabbage Slaw:

- 2 cups shredded cabbage
- 1/4 cup apple cider vinegar
- 1 tablespoon olive oil
- 1 teaspoon erythritol or sweetener of choice
- Salt and pepper to taste
- 2 tablespoons chopped fresh parsley

INSTRUCTIONS:

1. Combine paprika, cayenne pepper, garlic powder, salt, and pepper in a bowl. Rub the spice mixture over the pork ribs, ensuring they are well-coated. Let the ribs marinate for at least 1 hour or overnight in the refrigerator.
2. Preheat the oven to 300°F (150°C). Place the ribs on a baking sheet and drizzle with olive oil. Cover with foil and bake for about 1.5 hours, or until the meat is tender and pulls away from the bone.
3. While the ribs are baking, prepare the cabbage slaw by mixing the shredded cabbage, apple cider vinegar, olive oil, sweetener, salt, pepper, and parsley in a bowl. Toss well and refrigerate until ready to serve.
4. Once the ribs are done, let them rest for a few minutes before serving with the chilled cabbage slaw on the side.

NUTRITIONAL INFORMATION (PER SERVING):

Calories: 450 | Carbs: 5g | Fiber: 2g | Net Carbs: 3g
Protein: 30g | Fats: 35g

Meatloaf with Sun-Dried Tomatoes

Prep Time: 15 Minutes | **Cook Time:** 60 Minutes | **Serves:** 6

INGREDIENTS:

- 1.5 lbs ground beef
- 1/2 cup almond flour
- 1/2 cup sun-dried tomatoes, finely chopped
- 1 onion, finely chopped
- 2 cloves garlic, minced
- 1 egg, beaten
- 2 tablespoons Worcestershire sauce
- 1 teaspoon dried basil
- Salt and pepper to taste
- 1/4 cup low-carb ketchup or tomato paste for topping

INSTRUCTIONS:

1. Preheat your oven to 350°F (175°C). In a large bowl, mix together ground beef, almond flour, sun-dried tomatoes, onion, garlic, beaten egg, Worcestershire sauce, basil, salt, and pepper until well combined.
2. Transfer the mixture to a loaf pan or shape it into a loaf on a baking sheet lined with parchment paper.
3. Spread the low-carb ketchup or tomato paste over the top of the meatloaf.
4. Bake in the preheated oven for about 1 hour or until the meatloaf is cooked through and the top is slightly caramelized.
5. Let the meatloaf rest for 10 minutes before slicing and serving.

NUTRITIONAL INFORMATION (PER SERVING):

Calories: 350 | Carbs: 8g | Fiber: 2g | Net Carbs: 6g
Protein: 25g | Fats: 24g

Lamb Kofta with Tzatziki Sauce

Prep Time: 20 Minutes | **Cook Time:** 10 Minutes | **Serves:** 4

INGREDIENTS:

Ingredients for Lamb Kofta:

Ingredients for Tzatziki Sauce:

- 1 lb ground lamb
- 1 clove garlic, minced
- 1/4 cup onion, finely grated
- 2 cloves garlic, minced
- 2 tablespoons fresh parsley, finely chopped
- 1 teaspoon cumin
- 1/2 teaspoon coriander
- 1/2 teaspoon paprika
- Salt and pepper to taste
- 4 1 cup Greek yogurt, full-fat
- 1/2 cucumber, seeded and grated
- 1 tablespoon lemon juice
- 1 tablespoon olive oil
- 1 tablespoon fresh dill, chopped
- Salt to taste

INSTRUCTIONS:

1. In a bowl, combine all kofta ingredients. Mix well and form into small sausage shapes around skewers.
2. Grill koftas over medium heat, turning occasionally, until cooked through, about 8-10 minutes.
3. For the tzatziki sauce, mix Greek yogurt, grated cucumber, garlic, lemon juice, olive oil, and dill in a bowl. Season with salt and refrigerate until serving.
4. Serve lamb koftas with a side of tzatziki sauce.

NUTRITIONAL INFORMATION (PER SERVING):

Calories: 320 | Carbs: 6g | Fiber: 1g | Net Carbs: 5g
Protein: 22g | Fats: 24g

Beef and Eggplant Lasagna

Prep Time: 20 Minutes | **Cook Time:** 45 Minutes | **Serves:** 6

INGREDIENTS:

- 1 large eggplant, sliced lengthwise
- 1 lb ground beef
- 1/2 cup onion, chopped
- 2 cloves garlic, minced
- 1 can (14 oz) crushed tomatoes
- 1 egg
- 1 teaspoon Italian seasoning
- Salt and pepper to taste
- 1 1/2 cups ricotta cheese
- 1/2 cup Parmesan cheese, grated
- 1 cup mozzarella cheese, shredded

1. Preheat your oven to 375°F (190°C). Salt eggplant slices and let sit for 10 minutes, then rinse and pat dry.
2. In a skillet, cook ground beef, onion, and garlic until beef is browned. Add crushed tomatoes and Italian seasoning. Simmer for 10 minutes. Season with salt and pepper.
3. In a bowl, mix ricotta cheese, egg, and Parmesan cheese.
4. In a baking dish, layer eggplant slices, meat sauce, and ricotta mixture. Repeat layers and top with mozzarella cheese.
5. Bake for 30-35 minutes or until bubbly and golden. Let cool before serving.

NUTRITIONAL INFORMATION (PER SERVING):

Calories: 400 | Carbs: 12g | Fiber: 3g | Net Carbs: 9g
Protein: 28g | Fats: 28g

Pulled Pork Lettuce Wraps

Prep Time: 15 Minutes | **Cook Time:** 4 Hours |
Serves: 6

INGREDIENTS:

- 2 lbs pork shoulder
- Salt and pepper to taste
- 1 tablespoon olive oil
- 1/2 cup low-carb BBQ sauce
- 1 head of iceberg or butter lettuce, leaves separated
- 1/2 cup red onion, thinly sliced
- 1/2 cup cilantro, chopped

INSTRUCTIONS:

1. Season pork shoulder with salt and pepper. In a large pot, heat olive oil over medium heat and brown the pork on all sides.
2. Add 1 cup of water to the pot, cover, and simmer for about 4 hours or until the pork is tender and shreds easily.
3. Shred the pork using two forks and mix with low-carb BBQ sauce.
4. Place a spoonful of pulled pork on each lettuce leaf, top with sliced red onion and chopped cilantro.
5. Serve the lettuce wraps immediately.

NUTRITIONAL INFORMATION (PER SERVING):

Calories: 350 | Carbs: 45g | Fiber: 1g | Net Carbs: 4g
Protein: 25g | Fats: 25g

Beef and Pepper Fajita Bowls

Prep Time: 15 Minutes | **Cook Time:** 20 Minutes |
Serves: 4

INGREDIENTS:

- 1 lb beef flank steak, thinly sliced
- 2 bell peppers (any color), sliced
- 1 large onion, sliced
- 2 tablespoons olive oil
- 1 teaspoon chili powder
- 1 teaspoon cumin
- 1/2 teaspoon garlic powder
- Salt and pepper to taste
- 2 cups cauliflower rice, cooked
- Fresh cilantro and lime wedges for garnish

INSTRUCTIONS:

1. In a large skillet, heat 1 tablespoon olive oil over medium-high heat. Add the beef slices and season with chili powder, cumin, garlic powder, salt, and pepper. Cook until browned and cooked through, then set aside.
2. In the same skillet, add the remaining olive oil, bell peppers, and onion. Sauté until vegetables are tender and slightly charred.
3. Divide the cauliflower rice among four bowls. Top with the beef and sautéed peppers and onions.
4. Garnish with fresh cilantro and serve with lime wedges on the side.

NUTRITIONAL INFORMATION (PER SERVING):

Calories: 300 | Carbs: 10g | Fiber: 3g | Net Carbs: 7g
Protein: 25g | Fats: 18g

Grilled T-Bone Steak with Chimichurri

Prep Time: 15 Minutes | **Cook Time:** 10 Minutes |
Serves: 4

For the Chimichurri:

- 1 cup fresh parsley, finely chopped
- 1/4 cup olive oil
- 2 tablespoons red wine vinegar
- 2 garlic cloves, minced
- 1 teaspoon red pepper flakes
- Salt to taste
- 4 T-bone steaks
- Salt and pepper to taste

INSTRUCTIONS:

1. Season the T-bone steaks with salt and pepper, and let them come to room temperature.
2. Preheat your grill to high heat. Grill the steaks to your desired level of doneness, about 4-5 minutes per side for medium-rare.
3. For the chimichurri, combine parsley, olive oil, red wine vinegar, garlic, red pepper flakes, and salt in a bowl. Mix well.
4. Let the steaks rest for a few minutes after grilling. Serve each steak with a generous spoonful of chimichurri sauce on top.

NUTRITIONAL INFORMATION (PER SERVING):

Calories: 500 | Carbs: 2g | Fiber: 0.5g | Net Carbs: 1.5g
Protein: 45g | Fats: 35g

Pork Chops with Creamy Mushroom Sauce

Prep Time: 10 Minutes | **Cook Time:** 20 Minutes |
Serves: 4

INGREDIENTS:

- 4 pork chops
- Salt and pepper to taste
- 2 tablespoons olive oil
- 1 teaspoon thyme
- 1 cup mushrooms, sliced
- 1 clove garlic, minced
- 1/2 cup heavy cream
- 1/2 cup chicken broth

INSTRUCTIONS:

1. Season the pork chops with salt and pepper.
2. Heat olive oil in a large skillet over medium-high heat. Add pork chops and cook until golden and cooked through, about 5-7 minutes per side. Remove from the skillet and keep warm.
3. In the same skillet, add mushrooms and garlic. Cook until the mushrooms are soft.
4. Add chicken broth, heavy cream, and thyme to the skillet. Stir and scrape up any browned bits from the bottom of the pan. Simmer until the sauce thickens, about 5 minutes.
5. Return the pork chops to the skillet, coating them in the sauce. Cook for another 2-3 minutes.
6. Serve the pork chops with the creamy mushroom sauce spooned over the top.

NUTRITIONAL INFORMATION (PER SERVING):

Calories: 400 | Carbs: 3g | Fiber: 0.5g | Net Carbs: 2.5g
Protein: 30g | Fats: 30g

Beef Bulgogi with Kimchi

Prep Time: 15 Minutes | **Cook Time:** 10 Minutes |
Serves: 4

INGREDIENTS:

- 1 lb thinly sliced beef sirloin
- 1/4 cup soy sauce (or tamari for gluten-free)
- 2 tablespoons sesame oil
- 1 tablespoon erythritol or sweetener of choice
- 1 teaspoon grated ginger
- 2 cloves garlic, minced
- 1 tablespoon sesame seeds
- 1/2 onion, thinly sliced
- 1 green onion, chopped
- Salt and pepper to taste
- 1 cup kimchi for serving

INSTRUCTIONS:

1. In a bowl, combine soy sauce, sesame oil, sweetener, garlic, ginger, and sesame seeds to make the marinade.
2. Add the beef slices to the marinade, ensuring they are well coated. Cover and marinate in the refrigerator for at least 1 hour, or overnight for best flavor.
3. Heat a grill pan or skillet over medium-high heat. Remove beef from the marinade and cook with onion

slices until the beef is browned and cooked through, about 3-5 minutes.

4. Garnish with chopped green onions and serve with kimchi on the side.

Calories: 280 | Carbs: 5g | Fiber: 1g | Net Carbs: 4g
Protein: 25g | Fats: 18g

Lamb Stew with Turnips

Prep Time: 20 Minutes | **Cook Time:** 2 Hours | **Serves:** 6

INGREDIENTS:

- 2 lbs lamb stew meat, cut into chunks
- 3 tablespoons olive oil
- 4 cups beef broth
- 1 onion, chopped
- 2 cloves garlic, minced
- 2 cups turnips, peeled and diced
- 2 carrots, diced (optional, omit for lower carbs)
- 1 teaspoon rosemary
- 1 teaspoon thyme
- Salt and pepper to taste

INSTRUCTIONS:

1. In a large pot, heat olive oil over medium-high heat. Add lamb chunks and brown on all sides. Remove lamb and set aside.
2. In the same pot, add onion and garlic, cooking until softened.
3. Return lamb to the pot, add beef broth, rosemary, thyme, salt, and pepper. Bring to a boil, then reduce heat to low, cover, and simmer for 1.5 hours.
4. Add turnips and carrots (if using) to the pot. Continue to simmer for another 30 minutes, or until the vegetables and lamb are tender.
5. Adjust seasoning and serve hot.

NUTRITIONAL INFORMATION (PER SERVING):

Calories: 350 | Carbs: 6g | Fiber: 2g | Net Carbs: 4g
Protein: 40g | Fats: 18g

Italian Beef Braciole

Prep Time: 30 Minutes | **Cook Time:** 90 Minutes | **Serves:** 4

INGREDIENTS:

- 4 thin slices of beef round or flank steak
- 1/2 cup grated Parmesan cheese
- 2 cloves garlic, minced
- 2 tablespoons fresh parsley, chopped
- 1/4 cup almond flour
- Salt and pepper to taste
- 2 tablespoons olive oil
- 2 cups low-carb marinara sauce

INSTRUCTIONS:

1. Lay out the beef slices and season with salt and pepper. Sprinkle each with Parmesan cheese, garlic, parsley, and almond flour.
2. Roll up the beef slices tightly and secure with toothpicks.
3. In a large skillet, heat olive oil over medium-high heat. Brown the beef rolls on all sides.
4. Pour the marinara sauce over the beef rolls, cover, and simmer on low heat for 1 hour 30 minutes, or until the beef is tender.
5. Remove toothpicks, slice the rolls if desired, and serve with the sauce spooned over the top.

NUTRITIONAL INFORMATION (PER SERVING):

Calories: 380 | Carbs: 8g | Fiber: 2g | Net Carbs: 6g
Protein: 25g | Fats: 22g

Tenderloin with Crispy Shallots

Prep Time: 10 Minutes | **Cook Time:** 20 Minutes | **Serves:** 4

INGREDIENTS:

- 1 lb beef tenderloin, cut into 4 steaks
- Salt and pepper to taste
- 2 tablespoons olive oil
- 4 shallots, thinly sliced
- 1/2 cup beef broth
- 1 tablespoon butter
- Fresh thyme for garnish

1. Season the tenderloin steaks with salt and pepper.
2. Heat 1 tablespoon of olive oil in a skillet over medium-high heat. Add the steaks and cook to your desired level of doneness, about 4-5 minutes per side for medium-rare. Remove steaks and set aside to rest.
3. In the same skillet, add the remaining olive oil and shallots. Cook over medium heat, stirring occasionally, until shallots are golden and crispy.
4. Remove the shallots and set aside. Add beef broth to the skillet, scraping up any browned bits. Bring to a simmer and reduce by half.
5. Stir in the butter until melted and sauce is slightly thickened.
6. Serve the steaks with the sauce and top with crispy shallots. Garnish with fresh thyme.

NUTRITIONAL INFORMATION (PER SERVING):

Calories: 300 | Carbs: 4g | Fiber: 1g | Net Carbs: 3g
Protein: 30g | Fats: 18g

Pork Belly with Braised Cabbage

Prep Time: 15 Minutes | **Cook Time:** 2 Hours |
Serves: 4

INGREDIENTS:

- ❖ 1 lb pork belly, skin scored
- ❖ Salt and pepper to taste
- ❖ 1 tablespoon olive oil
- ❖ 1 head of cabbage, shredded
- ❖ 1 onion, sliced
- ❖ 1 apple, sliced (optional, omit for lower carbs)
- ❖ 1 cup chicken or vegetable broth
- ❖ 2 tablespoons apple cider vinegar
- ❖ 1 teaspoon caraway seeds (optional)

INSTRUCTIONS:

1. Preheat your oven to 350°F (175°C).
2. Season the pork belly with salt and pepper. Heat olive oil in an ovenproof skillet or Dutch oven and sear the pork belly on all sides until golden.
3. Remove the pork belly and set aside. In the same skillet, add the onion, cabbage, and apple (if using), cooking until softened.
4. Add broth, vinegar, and caraway seeds to the skillet. Bring to a simmer.
5. Braise for about 2 hours or until the pork belly is tender.
6. Serve the pork belly sliced with the braised cabbage on the side.

NUTRITIONAL INFORMATION (PER SERVING):

Calories: 500 | Carbs: 8g | Fiber: 3g | Net Carbs: 5g
Protein: 15g | Fats: 45g

Beef Short Ribs with Cauliflower Mash

Prep Time: 20 Minutes | **Cook Time:** 3 Hours |
Serves: 4

INGREDIENTS:

Ingredients for Beef Short Ribs:

- ❖ 2 lbs beef short ribs
- ❖ Salt and pepper to taste
- ❖ 2 tablespoons olive oil
- ❖ 1 onion, chopped
- ❖ 2 cloves garlic, minced
- ❖ 1 cup beef broth
- ❖ 1 cup red wine (optional, replace with more beef broth for no alcohol)

Ingredients for Cauliflower Mash:

- ❖ 1 large head cauliflower, cut into florets
- ❖ 2 tablespoons butter
- ❖ 1/4 cup heavy cream
- ❖ Salt and pepper to taste

INSTRUCTIONS:

1. Season the short ribs with salt and pepper. Heat olive oil in a large Dutch oven or pot over medium-high heat. Add the short ribs and brown on all sides. Remove and set aside.
2. In the same pot, add the onion and garlic, cooking until softened.
3. Return the short ribs to the pot. Add beef broth and red wine. Bring to a simmer, then cover and transfer to a preheated 325°F (163°C) oven.
4. Braise for about 2.5-3 hours or until the meat is tender and falls off the bone.
5. For the cauliflower mash, steam the cauliflower florets until tender. Blend in a food processor with butter, heavy cream, salt, and pepper until smooth.
6. Serve the short ribs with the cauliflower mash on the side.

Calories: 600 | Carbs: 12g | Fiber: 3g | Net Carbs: 9g
Protein: 40g | Fats: 45g

Gyro Salad with Lamb and Tzatziki

Prep Time: 20 Minutes | **Cook Time:** 15 Minutes |
Serves: 4

INGREDIENTS:

Ingredients for Gyro Salad:

- 1 lb lamb, thinly sliced
- 1 teaspoon oregano
- 2 cloves garlic, minced
- Salt and pepper to taste
- 1 tablespoon olive oil
- 4 cups mixed salad greens
- 1 cucumber, sliced
- 1/2 red onion, thinly sliced
- 1/2 cup cherry tomatoes, halved
- 1/4 cup Kalamata olives, pitted
- 1/4 cup feta cheese, crumbled

Ingredients for Tzatziki:

- 1 cup Greek yogurt, full-fat
- 1/2 cucumber, grated and drained
- 1 tablespoon lemon juice
- 1 tablespoon olive oil
- 1 clove garlic, minced
- Salt to taste
- Fresh dill, chopped

INSTRUCTIONS:

1. Season lamb with oregano, minced garlic, salt, and pepper.
2. Heat olive oil in a skillet over medium-high heat. Cook the lamb slices until browned and cooked through, about 3-5 minutes per side.
3. For the tzatziki, combine Greek yogurt, grated cucumber, lemon juice, olive oil, minced garlic, salt, and dill in a bowl. Mix until smooth.
4. Assemble the salad with mixed greens, cucumber, red onion, cherry tomatoes, olives, and crumbled feta. Top with cooked lamb.
5. Serve the gyro salad with tzatziki sauce on the side.

Calories: 350 | Carbs: 10g | Fiber: 2g | Net Carbs: 8g
Protein: 25g | Fats: 24g

Pork Loin Roast with Fennel and Rosemary

Prep Time: 15 Minutes | **Cook Time:** 1 Hour |
Serves: 6

INGREDIENTS:

- 2 lb pork loin roast
- 2 tablespoons olive oil
- 2 tablespoons fresh rosemary, chopped
- 2 cloves garlic, minced
- 1 bulb fennel, sliced
- Salt and pepper to taste

INSTRUCTIONS:

1. Preheat your oven to 375°F (190°C).
2. Rub the pork loin with olive oil, minced garlic, chopped rosemary, salt, and pepper.
3. Place the sliced fennel in a roasting pan and set the seasoned pork loin on top.
4. Roast in the preheated oven for about 1 hour or until the pork reaches an internal temperature of 145°F (63°C).
5. Let the pork rest for 10 minutes before slicing. Serve with roasted fennel.

Calories: 300 | Carbs: 5g | Fiber: 2g | Net Carbs: 3g
Protein: 40g | Fats: 14g

Beef Carpaccio with Arugula Salad

Prep Time: 15 Minutes | **Cook Time:** 0 Minute |
Serves: 4

INGREDIENTS:

- 1/2 lb beef tenderloin, trimmed and frozen for 2 hours
- 2 cups arugula
- 1/4 cup Parmesan cheese, shaved
- 1 tablespoon olive oil
- 1 tablespoon lemon juice
- Salt and pepper to taste
- Capers for garnish (optional)

INSTRUCTIONS:

1. Remove the beef tenderloin from the freezer and thinly slice it against the grain.
2. Arrange the beef slices on plates.
3. In a bowl, toss arugula with olive oil, lemon juice, salt, and pepper.
4. Place the arugula salad on top of the beef slices.
5. Garnish with shaved Parmesan and capers if desired.
6. Serve immediately.

Calories: 180 | Carbs: 1g | Fiber: 0.5g | Net Carbs: 0.5g
Protein: 20g | Fats: 10g

Lamb Curry with Coconut and Spinach

Prep Time: 20 Minutes | **Cook Time:** 1 Hour |
Serves: 4

INGREDIENTS:

- 1 lb lamb shoulder, cut into cubes
- 1 tablespoon coconut oil
- 1 large onion, finely chopped
- 2 cloves garlic, minced
- 1 tablespoon curry powder
- 1 teaspoon ground cumin
- 1 can (14 oz) coconut milk
- 2 cups spinach leaves, washed
- Salt and pepper to taste

INSTRUCTIONS:

1. Heat the coconut oil in a large pot over medium heat. Add the lamb cubes and brown on all sides, then remove and set aside.
2. In the same pot, add the onion and garlic, sautéing until softened.
3. Stir in the curry powder and cumin, cooking for another minute until fragrant.
4. Return the lamb to the pot and add the coconut milk. Bring to a simmer, then reduce the heat, cover, and cook for about 45 minutes or until the lamb is tender.
5. Stir in the spinach and cook until wilted. Season with salt and pepper to taste.
6. Serve hot, ideally over cauliflower rice for a complete low-carb meal.

Calories: 400 | Carbs: 8g | Fiber: 2g | Net Carbs: 6g
Protein: 25g | Fats: 32g

Ground Beef Tacos

Prep Time: 15 Minutes | **Cook Time:** 10 Minutes |
Serves: 4

INGREDIENTS:

- 1 lb ground beef
- 1 tablespoon olive oil
- 1/2 onion, finely chopped
- 2 cloves garlic, minced
- 1 tablespoon taco seasoning
- 8 low-carb tortillas
- **Toppings:** shredded lettuce, diced tomatoes, shredded cheese, avocado slices, and sour cream

INSTRUCTIONS:

1. Heat the olive oil in a skillet over medium heat. Add the onion and garlic, sautéing until softened.
2. Add the ground beef and taco seasoning, cooking until the beef is browned and cooked through.
3. Warm the low-carb tortillas according to package instructions.
4. Assemble the tacos by placing a spoonful of the beef mixture onto each tortilla, then top with lettuce, tomatoes, cheese, avocado, and a dollop of sour cream.
5. Serve immediately.

Calories: 300 | Carbs: 6g | Fiber: 1g | Net Carbs: 5g
Protein: 20g | Fats: 22g

Bacon and Spinach Stuffed Pork

Prep Time: 30 Minutes | **Cook Time:** 45 Minutes |
Serves: 4

INGREDIENTS:

- 1 pork tenderloin (about 1.5 lbs)
- 1 tablespoon olive oil
- 4 slices of bacon, cooked and crumbled

- ❖ 2 cups fresh spinach, wilted and squeezed dry
- ❖ 1/2 cup feta cheese, crumbled
- ❖ Salt and pepper to taste
- ❖ Toothpicks or kitchen twine for securing

INSTRUCTIONS:

1. Preheat your oven to 375°F (190°C).
2. Butterfly the pork tenderloin by slicing it lengthwise, being careful not to cut all the way through. Open it up like a book and flatten it with a meat mallet.
3. Layer the inside of the tenderloin with spinach, crumbled bacon, and feta cheese. Roll up the tenderloin and secure it with toothpicks or kitchen twine.
4. Season the outside of the tenderloin with salt and pepper. Heat the olive oil in a skillet over medium-high heat and sear the tenderloin on all sides.
5. Transfer the seared tenderloin to a baking dish and roast in the preheated oven for 30-35 minutes, or until the internal temperature reaches 145°F (63°C).
6. Let the tenderloin rest for 10 minutes before slicing and serving.

Zoodles Carbonara

Prep Time: 15 Minutes | **Cook Time:** 10 Minutes |
Serves: 4

INGREDIENTS:

- ❖ 4 medium zucchinis, spiralized into zoodles
- ❖ 2 teaspoons olive oil
- ❖ 4 slices of bacon, diced
- ❖ 2 garlic cloves, minced
- ❖ 2 large eggs
- ❖ 1/2 cup grated Parmesan cheese
- ❖ Salt and pepper, to taste
- ❖ Fresh parsley, chopped (for garnish)

INSTRUCTIONS:

1. Heat olive oil in a large pan over medium heat. Add bacon and cook until crispy. Add garlic and sauté for 1 minute.
2. Add zoodles to the pan and sauté for 2-3 minutes until tender. Remove from heat.
3. In a bowl, whisk together eggs and Parmesan cheese. Pour this mixture over the zoodles in the pan, tossing quickly to coat and gently cook the eggs with the residual heat. Season with salt and pepper.
4. Serve immediately, garnished with fresh parsley.

Beef Taco Salad with Avocado

Prep Time: 20 Minutes | **Cook Time:** 10 Minutes |
Serves: 4

INGREDIENTS:

- ❖ 1 lb lean ground beef
- ❖ 1 tablespoon taco seasoning (sugar-free)
- ❖ 1/4 cup water
- ❖ 4 cups mixed salad greens
- ❖ 1/2 cup cherry tomatoes, halved
- ❖ 1 large avocado, diced
- ❖ 1/4 cup shredded cheddar cheese
- ❖ 1/4 cup sour cream
- ❖ 2 tablespoons cilantro, chopped
- ❖ Lime wedges, for serving

INSTRUCTIONS:

1. In a skillet over medium heat, cook the ground beef until browned. Drain excess fat.
2. Stir in taco seasoning and water. Simmer for 5 minutes until the water is absorbed. Remove from heat.
3. In a large bowl, toss salad greens, avocado, and cherry tomatoes. Divide among serving plates.
4. Top salads with cooked taco meat, shredded cheese, and a dollop of sour cream.
5. Garnish with cilantro and serve with lime wedges on the side.

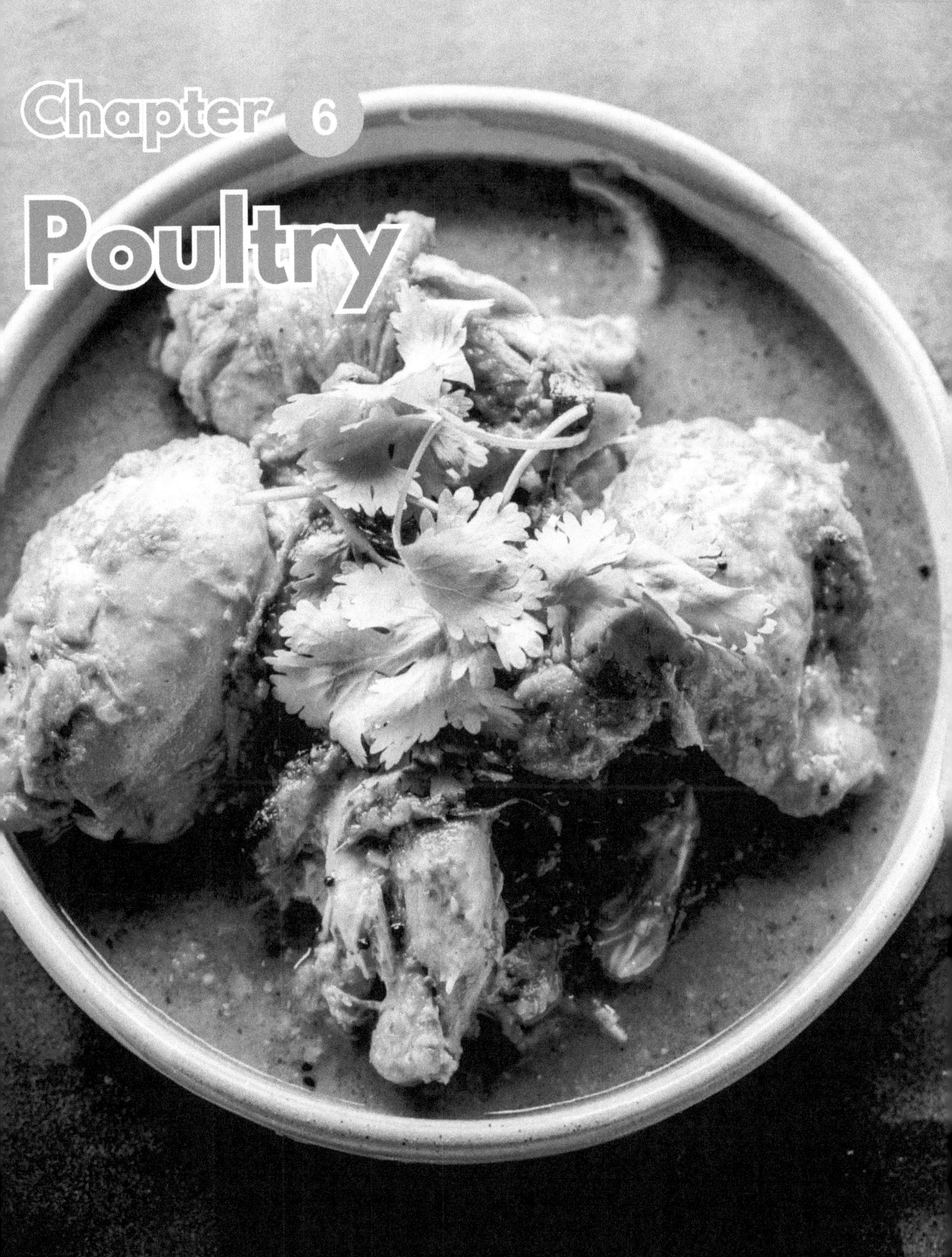

Chapter 6
Poultry

Grilled Chicken with Avocado Salsa

Prep Time: 15 Minutes | **Cook Time:** 20 Minutes | **Serves:** 4

INGREDIENTS:

Ingredients for Grilled Chicken:

* 4 boneless, skinless chicken breasts
* 2 tablespoons olive oil
* 1 teaspoon chili powder
* 1 teaspoon garlic powder
* Salt and pepper to taste

Ingredients for Avocado Salsa:

* 2 ripe avocados, diced
* 1 small red onion, finely chopped
* 1 tomato, diced
* Juice of 1 lime
* 2 tablespoons cilantro, chopped
* Salt to taste

INSTRUCTIONS:

1. Preheat your grill to medium-high heat.
2. Rub the chicken breasts with olive oil and season with chili powder, garlic powder, salt, and pepper.
3. Grill the chicken for about 10 minutes on each side or until fully cooked and juices run clear.
4. While the chicken is grilling, combine diced avocados, chopped red onion, diced tomato, lime juice, cilantro, and salt in a bowl to make the salsa. Mix gently to combine.
5. Serve the grilled chicken topped with a generous portion of avocado salsa.

NUTRITIONAL INFORMATION (PER SERVING):

Calories: 350 | Carbs: 10g | Fiber: 5g | Net Carbs: 5g
Protein: 30g | Fats: 22g

Turkey Zucchini Meatballs

Prep Time: 20 Minutes | **Cook Time:** 25 Minutes | **Serves:** 4

INGREDIENTS:

* 1 lb ground turkey
* 1/4 cup almond flour
* 1 cup zucchini, grated and squeezed dry
* 1 egg
* 2 cloves garlic, minced
* 1 teaspoon Italian seasoning
* Salt and pepper to taste
* 1 cup low-carb marinara sauce

INSTRUCTIONS:

1. Preheat your oven to 375°F (190°C). Line a baking sheet with parchment paper.
2. In a large bowl, combine ground turkey, grated zucchini, almond flour, egg, minced garlic, Italian seasoning, salt, and pepper. Mix until well combined.
3. Form the mixture into meatballs and place them on the prepared baking sheet.
4. Bake for 20-25 minutes or until the meatballs are cooked through.
5. Warm the marinara sauce in a saucepan and serve with the meatballs.

NUTRITIONAL INFORMATION (PER SERVING):

Calories: 240 | Carbs: 6g | Fiber: 2g | Net Carbs: 4g
Protein: 28g | Fats: 12g

Chicken Caesar Salad Wraps

Prep Time: 15 Minutes | **Cook Time:** 10 Minutes | **Serves:** 4

INGREDIENTS:

* 2 chicken breasts, grilled and sliced
* 4 low-carb tortillas or large lettuce leaves
* 4 cups romaine lettuce, chopped
* 1/2 cup Caesar dressing, low-carb
* 1/4 cup Parmesan cheese, grated
* Salt and pepper to taste

INSTRUCTIONS:

1. If using chicken breasts, grill the chicken seasoned with salt and pepper until fully cooked, then slice thinly.
2. Lay out the low-carb tortillas or large lettuce leaves on a flat surface.
3. Toss the chopped romaine lettuce with Caesar dressing and grated Parmesan cheese.
4. Divide the Caesar salad among the tortillas or lettuce

leaves, topping with slices of grilled chicken.

5. Roll up the tortillas or lettuce leaves to enclose the filling and serve immediately.

Calories: 300 | Carbs: 6g | Fiber: 2g | Net Carbs: 4g
Protein: 25g | Fats: 20g

Spicy Buffalo Cauliflower Bites

Prep Time: 15 Minutes | **Cook Time:** 25 Minutes |
Serves: 4

INGREDIENTS:

- 1 large head cauliflower, cut into bite-sized florets
- 1 teaspoon garlic powder
- Salt and pepper to taste
- 1 tablespoon olive oil
- 1/2 cup hot sauce (e.g., Frank's Red Hot)
- 1 tablespoon unsalted butter, melted

INSTRUCTIONS:

1. Preheat your oven to 425°F (220°C) and line a baking sheet with parchment paper.
2. Toss the cauliflower florets with olive oil, salt, and pepper, and spread them out on the baking sheet.
3. Roast in the oven for about 20 minutes or until the cauliflower starts to become tender and slightly browned.
4. In a small bowl, mix together the hot sauce, melted butter, and garlic powder.
5. Remove the cauliflower from the oven and toss with the hot sauce mixture until well coated.
6. Return the cauliflower to the oven and roast for an additional 5 minutes.
7. Serve hot, garnished with fresh chopped parsley if desired.

NUTRITIONAL INFORMATION (PER SERVING):

Calories: 100 | Carbs: 8g | Fiber: 3g | Net Carbs: 5g
Protein: 3g | Fats: 7g

Duck Breast with Red Wine Sauce

Prep Time: 15 Minutes | **Cook Time:** 30 Minutes |
Serves: 2

INGREDIENTS:

- 2 duck breasts, skin on
- Salt and pepper to taste
- 1/2 cup red wine
- 1/4 cup chicken broth
- 1 tablespoon unsalted butter
- 1 teaspoon fresh thyme, chopped

INSTRUCTIONS:

1. Score the skin of the duck breasts in a diamond pattern and season with salt and pepper.
2. Heat a skillet over medium heat and place the duck breasts skin-side down. Cook for about 6-8 minutes until the skin is crispy and golden.
3. Flip the duck breasts and cook for an additional 5-7 minutes for medium-rare. Remove and let rest.
4. In the same skillet, add red wine and chicken broth, scraping up the browned bits from the bottom. Reduce by half.
5. Stir in the butter and thyme until the sauce thickens slightly.
6. Slice the duck breasts and serve with the red wine sauce drizzled over the top.

NUTRITIONAL INFORMATION (PER SERVING):

Calories: 400 | Carbs: 2g | Fiber: 0g | Net Carbs: 2g
Protein: 30g | Fats: 28g

Chicken and Asparagus Lemon Stir Fry

Prep Time: 15 Minutes | **Cook Time:** 15 Minutes |
Serves: 4

INGREDIENTS:

- 1 lb chicken breast, thinly sliced
- 1 lb asparagus, trimmed and cut into 1-inch pieces
- 1 lemon, zest and juice
- 2 tablespoons olive oil, divided
- 2 cloves garlic, minced
- Salt and pepper to taste

1. Heat 1 tablespoon of olive oil in a large skillet over medium-high heat. Add the chicken and season with salt and pepper. Stir-fry until the chicken is cooked through, about 5-7 minutes. Remove and set aside.
2. In the same skillet, add the remaining olive oil and asparagus. Stir-fry until tender-crisp, about 3-4 minutes.
3. Add the garlic and lemon zest, cooking for an additional minute until fragrant.
4. Return the chicken to the skillet, add lemon juice, and toss to combine. Heat through.
5. Serve hot, garnished with additional lemon zest if desired.

NUTRITIONAL INFORMATION (PER SERVING):

Calories: 250 | Carbs: 6g | Fiber: 2g | Net Carbs: 4g
Protein: 30g | Fats: 12g

Shredded Buffalo Chicken

Prep Time: 10 Minutes | **Cook Time:** 4 Hours |
Serves: 4

INGREDIENTS:

- 1 lb chicken breasts
- 1/4 cup chicken broth
- 1/2 cup buffalo sauce
- 2 tablespoons unsalted butter
- Salt and pepper to taste
- Optional for serving: celery sticks, low-carb blue cheese dressing

INSTRUCTIONS:

1. Place chicken breasts in a slow cooker. Season with salt and pepper.
2. Pour buffalo sauce and chicken broth over the chicken. Add butter on top.
3. Cover and cook on low for 4 hours in the slow cooker or simmer covered on the stovetop for 1 hour until chicken is tender and fully cooked.
4. Shred the chicken with two forks and mix well with the sauce.
5. Serve the shredded buffalo chicken with celery sticks and low-carb blue cheese dressing on the side if desired.

NUTRITIONAL INFORMATION (PER SERVING):

Calories: 220 | Carbs: 1g | Fiber: 0g | Net Carbs: 1g
Protein: 25g | Fats: 12g

Turkey and Spinach Stuffed Mushrooms

Prep Time: 20 Minutes | **Cook Time:** 20 Minutes |
Serves: 4

INGREDIENTS:

- 16 large mushrooms, stems removed
- 1/2 lb ground turkey
- 1 cup spinach, chopped
- 1/4 cup onion, finely chopped
- 2 cloves garlic, minced
- 1/4 cup grated Parmesan cheese
- 2 tablespoons olive oil
- Salt and pepper to taste

INSTRUCTIONS:

1. Preheat your oven to 375°F (190°C).
2. Heat 1 tablespoon olive oil in a skillet over medium heat. Cook the turkey, onion, and garlic until the turkey is browned.
3. Stir in the spinach until wilted. Remove from heat and mix in the Parmesan cheese. Season with salt and pepper.
4. Brush the mushroom caps with the remaining olive oil and place them on a baking sheet.
5. Stuff each mushroom cap with the turkey and spinach mixture.
6. Bake for 20 minutes or until the mushrooms are tender.
7. Serve warm.

NUTRITIONAL INFORMATION (PER SERVING):

Calories: 180 | Carbs: 5g | Fiber: 1g | Net Carbs: 4g
Protein: 15g | Fats: 12g

Balsamic Glazed Chicken Drumsticks

Prep Time: 10 Minutes | **Cook Time:** 40 Minutes |
Serves: 4

- 8 chicken drumsticks
- Salt and pepper to taste
- 1/2 cup balsamic vinegar
- 2 tablespoons olive oil
- 2 cloves garlic, minced
- 1 tablespoon erythritol or sweetener of choice
- 1 teaspoon dried rosemary or thyme

INSTRUCTIONS:

1. Preheat your oven to 400°F (200°C).
2. Season the drumsticks with salt and pepper and place them in a baking dish.
3. In a saucepan, combine balsamic vinegar, olive oil, garlic, sweetener, and herbs. Simmer until the mixture reduces by half and thickens into a glaze.
4. Brush the glaze over the chicken drumsticks, reserving some for basting.
5. Bake for 40 minutes, basting with the remaining glaze halfway through cooking, until the chicken is cooked through and the glaze is caramelized.
6. Serve hot.

NUTRITIONAL INFORMATION (PER SERVING):

Calories: 300 | Carbs: 6g | Fiber: 0g | Net Carbs: 6g

Protein: 24g | Fats: 20g

Grain-Free Parmesan Chicken

Prep Time: 15 Minutes | **Cook Time:** 25 Minutes |
Serves: 4

INGREDIENTS:

- 4 boneless, skinless chicken breasts
- 1/2 cup grated Parmesan cheese
- 1/4 cup almond flour
- 1 teaspoon garlic powder
- 1/2 teaspoon paprika
- Salt and pepper to taste
- 2 tablespoons olive oil
- 1 egg, beaten

INSTRUCTIONS:

1. Preheat your oven to 375°F (190°C).
2. In a shallow dish, combine grated Parmesan, almond flour, garlic powder, paprika, salt, and pepper.
3. Dip each chicken breast in the beaten egg, then coat with the Parmesan mixture.
4. Heat olive oil in a large oven-proof skillet over medium-high heat. Add the chicken and sear for 2-3 minutes on each side until golden.
5. Transfer the skillet to the oven and bake for 20 minutes, or until the chicken is cooked through and the coating is crispy.
6. Serve hot, garnished with fresh herbs if desired.

NUTRITIONAL INFORMATION (PER SERVING):

Calories: 320 | Carbs: 2g | Fiber: 1g | Net Carbs: 1g

Protein: 35g | Fats: 18g

Pesto Chicken Stuffed Bell Peppers

Prep Time: 20 Minutes | **Cook Time:** 30 Minutes |
Serves: 4

INGREDIENTS:

- 4 bell peppers, halved and seeds removed
- 2 cups cooked and shredded chicken breast
- 1/2 cup pesto sauce
- 1 cup mozzarella cheese, shredded
- 1/4 cup sun-dried tomatoes, chopped (optional)
- Salt and pepper to taste

INSTRUCTIONS:

1. Preheat your oven to 350°F (175°C).
2. In a bowl, mix the shredded chicken with pesto sauce, half of the mozzarella cheese, sun-dried tomatoes (if using), salt, and pepper.
3. Stuff each bell pepper half with the chicken mixture and place them in a baking dish.
4. Top with the remaining mozzarella cheese.
5. Bake for 30 minutes, or until the peppers are tender and the cheese is bubbly and golden.
6. Serve hot, garnished with fresh basil if desired.

NUTRITIONAL INFORMATION (PER SERVING):

Calories: 400 | Carbs: 9g | Fiber: 2g | Net Carbs: 7g

Protein: 30g | Fats: 27g

Chicken Alfredo Spaghetti Squash

Prep Time: 15 Minutes | **Cook Time:** 45 Minutes | **Serves:** 4

INGREDIENTS:

- 1 large spaghetti squash, halved and seeds removed
- 2 tablespoons olive oil
- 2 cups cooked chicken breast, shredded
- 1 cup Alfredo sauce, low-carb
- 1/2 cup Parmesan cheese, grated
- 1/4 cup fresh parsley, chopped
- Salt and pepper to taste

INSTRUCTIONS:

1. Preheat your oven to 400°F (200°C). Brush the cut sides of the spaghetti squash with olive oil and season with salt and pepper.
2. Place the squash cut-side down on a baking sheet and roast for 30-40 minutes, or until tender.
3. Use a fork to scrape the squash strands into a bowl.
4. In a large skillet, combine the spaghetti squash strands, shredded chicken, and Alfredo sauce. Cook over medium heat until heated through.
5. Serve the mixture in the squash shells or a serving dish, topped with grated Parmesan and fresh parsley.

NUTRITIONAL INFORMATION (PER SERVING):

Calories: 350 | Carbs: 8g | Fiber: 2g | Net Carbs: 6g | Protein: 25g | Fats: 24g

Turkey Bacon and Avocado Club

Prep Time: 10 Minutes | **Cook Time:** 10 Minutes | **Serves:** 4

INGREDIENTS:

- 8 slices turkey bacon
- 1 large avocado, sliced
- 1/2 cup mayonnaise, low-carb
- 8 large lettuce leaves (Romaine or Iceberg)
- 1 tomato, sliced
- Salt and pepper to taste

INSTRUCTIONS:

1. Cook the turkey bacon in a skillet over medium heat until crispy, about 5 minutes per side. Drain on paper towels.
2. Spread a thin layer of low-carb mayonnaise on one side of 4 lettuce leaves.
3. Top each with 2 slices of cooked turkey bacon, avocado slices, and tomato slices. Season with salt and pepper.
4. Cover with another lettuce leaf, creating a sandwich. Secure with toothpicks if necessary.
5. Serve immediately.

NUTRITIONAL INFORMATION (PER SERVING):

Calories: 300 | Carbs: 6g | Fiber: 3g | Net Carbs: 3g | Protein: 10g | Fats: 26g

Chicken Shawarma Salad

Prep Time: 20 Minutes | **Cook Time:** 20 Minutes | **Serves:** 4

INGREDIENTS:

Ingredients for Chicken:

- 1 lb chicken thighs, boneless and skinless
- 2 tablespoons olive oil
- 1 tablespoon shawarma spice blend
- Juice of 1 lemon
- Salt to taste

Ingredients for Salad:

- 4 cups mixed greens
- 1 cucumber, diced
- 1/2 red onion, thinly sliced
- 1/4 cup fresh parsley, chopped
- 2 tablespoons olive oil
- 1 tablespoon lemon juice
- Salt and pepper to taste

INSTRUCTIONS:

1. Marinate the chicken thighs in olive oil, shawarma spice blend, lemon juice, and salt for at least 1 hour or overnight in the refrigerator.
2. Preheat the grill or a grill pan over medium-high heat. Grill the chicken for about 10 minutes per side or until fully cooked and slightly charred.
3. Let the chicken rest for a few minutes, then slice thinly.
4. Toss the mixed greens, cucumber, red onion, and

parsley with olive oil, lemon juice, salt, and pepper.

5. Divide the salad among plates and top with sliced chicken shawarma.
6. Serve immediately.

Calories: 350 | Carbs: 6g | Fiber: 2g | Net Carbs: 4g
Protein: 25g | Fats: 25g

Thai Turkey Lettuce Wraps

Prep Time: 15 Minutes | **Cook Time:** 15 Minutes
Serves: 4

INGREDIENTS:

- 1 lb ground turkey
- 1 tablespoon olive oil
- 2 cloves garlic, minced
- 1 tablespoon ginger, minced
- 1 red bell pepper, diced
- 1/4 cup green onions, chopped
- 2 tablespoons soy sauce (or tamari for gluten-free)
- 1/4 cup cilantro, chopped
- 1 tablespoon fish sauce
- 1 tablespoon lime juice
- 1 teaspoon erythritol or sweetener of choice
- 1 teaspoon crushed red pepper flakes (optional)
- 8 large lettuce leaves (Butter or Romaine)

INSTRUCTIONS:

1. Heat olive oil in a large skillet over medium heat. Add garlic and ginger, sautéing until fragrant.
2. Add ground turkey to the skillet, breaking it up with a spoon, and cook until browned.
3. Stir in diced red bell pepper, green onions, and cilantro. Cook for an additional 5 minutes.
4. Add soy sauce, fish sauce, lime juice, sweetener, and red pepper flakes (if using). Cook for another 2-3 minutes, allowing the flavors to blend.
5. Spoon the turkey mixture into lettuce leaves and serve as wraps.

Calories: 250 | Carbs: 6g | Fiber: 1g | Net Carbs: 5g
Protein: 25g | Fats: 14g

Chicken Piccata with Artichokes

Prep Time: 20 Minutes | **Cook Time:** 25 Minutes
Serves: 4

INGREDIENTS:

- 4 boneless, skinless chicken breasts, pounded thin
- Salt and pepper to taste
- 2 tablespoons olive oil
- 1/2 cup chicken broth
- 1/4 cup lemon juice
- 1 can (14 oz) artichoke hearts, drained and quartered
- 2 tablespoons capers, rinsed
- 2 tablespoons unsalted butter
- Fresh parsley, chopped for garnish

INSTRUCTIONS:

1. Season the chicken breasts with salt and pepper.
2. Heat olive oil in a large skillet over medium-high heat. Add the chicken and cook until golden and cooked through, about 3-4 minutes per side. Remove chicken and set aside.
3. To the same skillet, add chicken broth and lemon juice, scraping up any browned bits. Add artichoke hearts and capers. Simmer until the sauce is slightly reduced, about 5 minutes.
4. Stir in the butter until melted and the sauce is slightly thickened.
5. Return the chicken to the skillet, coating it in the sauce. Heat through.
6. Serve the chicken topped with the sauce, garnished with fresh parsley.

Calories: 280 | Carbs: 4g | Fiber: 1g | Net Carbs: 3g
Protein: 25g | Fats: 18g

Ground Turkey Tetrazzini

Prep Time: 15 Minutes | **Cook Time:** 30 Minutes | **Serves:** 4

INGREDIENTS:

- 1 lb ground turkey
- 1 tablespoon olive oil
- 1/2 onion, chopped
- 2 cloves garlic, minced
- 1/2 cup chicken broth
- 1 cup heavy cream
- 1/2 cup grated Parmesan cheese
- 2 cups zucchini noodles or spaghetti squash strands
- Salt and pepper to taste
- Fresh parsley, chopped for garnish

INSTRUCTIONS:

1. Heat olive oil in a large skillet over medium heat. Add the ground turkey, onion, and garlic, cooking until the turkey is browned.
2. Stir in chicken broth and heavy cream, bringing to a simmer. Add the Parmesan cheese, stirring until melted and the sauce is thickened.
3. Add the zucchini noodles or spaghetti squash, tossing to coat in the sauce. Cook until heated through, about 5 minutes.
4. Season with salt and pepper to taste.
5. Serve garnished with fresh parsley.

NUTRITIONAL INFORMATION (PER SERVING):

Calories: 350 | Carbs: 6g | Fiber: 1g | Net Carbs: 5g
Protein: 28g | Fats: 24g

Roast Duck with Orange and Ginger

Prep Time: 20 Minutes | **Cook Time:** 2 Hours | **Serves:** 4

INGREDIENTS:

- 1 whole duck, about 4-5 lbs
- Salt and pepper to taste
- 2 oranges, quartered
- 2-inch piece of ginger, sliced
- 1/4 cup soy sauce (or tamari for gluten-free)
- 2 tablespoons honey (optional, omit for lower carbs)
- 1 tablespoon olive oil

INSTRUCTIONS:

1. Preheat your oven to 350°F (175°C). Season the duck inside and out with salt and pepper.
2. Stuff the duck cavity with orange quarters and ginger slices.
3. In a small bowl, mix together soy sauce, honey (if using), and olive oil. Brush this mixture over the duck.
4. Place the duck breast side up on a rack in a roasting pan. Roast for about 2 hours, or until the skin is crispy and the meat is fully cooked, basting occasionally with the pan juices.
5. Let the duck rest for 10 minutes before carving.
6. Serve with additional orange slices and garnish with fresh herbs if desired.

NUTRITIONAL INFORMATION (PER SERVING):

Calories: 500 | Carbs: 3g | Fiber: 0g | Net Carbs: 3g
Protein: 40g | Fats: 36g

Rosemary Chicken with Potato and Green Beans

Prep Time: 15 Minutes | **Cook Time:** 35 Minutes | **Serves:** 4

INGREDIENTS:

- 4 boneless, skinless chicken breasts
- 2 tablespoons olive oil
- 2 teaspoons fresh rosemary, chopped
- Salt and pepper to taste
- 1 lb green beans, trimmed
- 1 lb small potatoes, halved (use a low-carb alternative like radishes for a lower carb option)
- 2 cloves garlic, minced

INSTRUCTIONS:

1. Preheat your oven to 375°F (190°C).
2. In a large bowl, toss the chicken breasts with 1 tablespoon olive oil, rosemary, salt, and pepper.
3. In another bowl, toss the green beans and potatoes (or radishes) with the remaining olive oil, garlic, salt, and pepper.

4. Spread the green beans and potatoes in a single layer on a baking sheet. Place the seasoned chicken breasts on top.
5. Roast in the preheated oven for about 35 minutes, or until the chicken is cooked through and the vegetables are tender.
6. Serve hot, garnished with additional rosemary if desired.

NUTRITIONAL INFORMATION (PER SERVING):

Calories: 320 | Carbs: 10g | Fiber: 3g | Net Carbs: 7g
Protein: 30g | Fats: 18g

Baked Chicken Stuffed with Collard Greens

Prep Time: 20 Minutes | **Cook Time:** 30 Minutes |
Serves: 4

INGREDIENTS:

- 1 bunch collard greens, stems removed and chopped
- 1 tablespoon olive oil
- 1/2 cup ricotta cheese
- 2 cloves garlic, minced
- 4 boneless, skinless chicken breasts
- Salt and pepper to taste

INSTRUCTIONS:

1. Preheat your oven to 375°F (190°C).
2. In a skillet, sauté the collard greens and garlic in olive oil until the greens are wilted. Season with salt and pepper. Let cool slightly, then mix in the ricotta cheese.
3. Cut a pocket into the side of each chicken breast. Stuff the collard green mixture into each pocket and secure with toothpicks if needed.
4. Season the outside of the chicken breasts with salt and pepper.
5. Place the stuffed chicken breasts in a baking dish and bake for about 30 minutes, or until the chicken is cooked through.
6. Serve hot.

NUTRITIONAL INFORMATION (PER SERVING):

Calories: 250 | Carbs: 3g | Fiber: 1g | Net Carbs: 2g
Protein: 35g | Fats: 11g

Chicken Fajita Stuffed Peppers

Prep Time: 20 Minutes | **Cook Time:** 25 Minutes |
Serves: 4

INGREDIENTS:

- 4 large bell peppers, halved and seeded
- 1 tablespoon olive oil
- 1 teaspoon cumin
- 1 onion, thinly sliced
- 1/2 cup sliced bell peppers (various colors)
- 1 lb chicken breast, thinly sliced
- 1 teaspoon chili powder
- Salt and pepper to taste
- 1/2 cup shredded cheddar cheese

INSTRUCTIONS:

1. Start by preheating your oven to 375°F (190°C).
2. In a skillet, heat the olive oil over medium heat. Add the chicken, onion, and sliced bell peppers. Season with chili powder, cumin, salt, and pepper. Cook until the chicken is browned and the vegetables are tender.
3. Place the halved bell peppers in a baking dish, cut-side up. Spoon the chicken and vegetable mixture into each bell pepper half.
4. Top each stuffed pepper with shredded cheddar cheese.
5. Bake in the preheated oven for about 25 minutes, or until the peppers are tender and the cheese is melted and bubbly.
6. Serve hot.

NUTRITIONAL INFORMATION (PER SERVING):

Calories: 300 | Carbs: 10g | Fiber: 3g | Net Carbs: 7g
Protein: 30g | Fats: 16g

Lemon and Herb Roasted Chicken

Prep Time: 15 Minutes | **Cook Time:** 20 Minutes |
Serves: 4

INGREDIENTS:

- 1 whole chicken (about 4 lbs)
- 2 tablespoons olive oil
- 2 lemons, one juiced and one sliced
- 2 tablespoons fresh herbs (such as rosemary, thyme, and parsley), chopped

❖ 4 cloves garlic, minced
❖ Salt and pepper to taste

INSTRUCTIONS:

1. Preheat your oven to 375°F (190°C).
2. Rinse the chicken and pat dry with paper towels. Season the cavity with salt and pepper, and stuff with lemon slices and half of the chopped herbs.
3. In a small bowl, mix together olive oil, lemon juice, remaining herbs, garlic, salt, and pepper.
4. Rub the herb mixture all over the chicken, ensuring it's well coated.
5. Place the chicken in a roasting pan and roast in the preheated oven for about 1 hour and 20 minutes, or until the juices run clear and a thermometer inserted into the thickest part of the thigh reads 165°F (74°C).
6. Let the chicken rest for 10 minutes before carving. Serve with additional lemon slices and fresh herbs if desired.

NUTRITIONAL INFORMATION (PER SERVING):

Calories: 400 | Carbs: 3g | Fiber: 1g | Net Carbs: 2g
Protein: 35g | Fats: 28g

Cast Iron Hot Chicken

Prep Time: 20 Minutes | **Cook Time:** 30 Minutes |
Serves: 4

INGREDIENTS:

❖ 8 chicken thighs, bone-in and skin-on
❖ 1 teaspoon cayenne pepper (adjust to taste)
❖ 1 cup buttermilk (for a low-carb version, use 1 cup almond milk mixed with 1 tablespoon vinegar)
❖ 1 teaspoon garlic powder
❖ Salt and pepper to taste
❖ 2 tablespoons hot sauce
❖ 2 tablespoons olive oil
❖ 1 tablespoon paprika

INSTRUCTIONS:

1. In a large bowl, mix together buttermilk, hot sauce, paprika, cayenne pepper, garlic powder, salt, and pepper. Add chicken thighs, ensuring they're fully coated. Marinate for at least 1 hour or overnight in the refrigerator.
2. Preheat your oven to 425°F (220°C).
3. Heat olive oil in a large cast-iron skillet over medium-high heat. Remove chicken from the marinade and place skin-side down in the skillet. Cook until the skin is crispy, about 5 minutes.
4. Flip the chicken thighs and transfer the skillet to the preheated oven. Roast until the chicken is cooked through, about 25 minutes.
5. Serve hot, garnished with additional hot sauce if desired.

NUTRITIONAL INFORMATION (PER SERVING):

Calories: 450 | Carbs: 2g | Fiber: 0.5g | Net Carbs: 1.5g
Protein: 35g | Fats: 34g

Turkey and Vegetable Skillet

Prep Time: 10 Minutes | **Cook Time:** 20 Minutes |
Serves: 4

INGREDIENTS:

❖ 1 lb ground turkey
❖ 1 onion, diced
❖ 1 tablespoon olive oil
❖ 2 cloves garlic, minced
❖ 1 bell pepper, diced
❖ 1 teaspoon Italian seasoning
❖ 1 zucchini, diced
❖ 1 cup cherry tomatoes, halved
❖ Salt and pepper to taste

INSTRUCTIONS:

1. Heat olive oil in a large skillet over medium heat. Add the onion and garlic, cooking until softened.
2. Add the ground turkey to the skillet, breaking it apart with a spoon. Cook until browned.
3. Stir in the bell pepper, zucchini, and cherry tomatoes. Season with Italian seasoning, salt, and pepper.
4. Cook, stirring occasionally, until the vegetables are tender, about 10 minutes.
5. Serve hot, garnished with fresh herbs if desired.

NUTRITIONAL INFORMATION (PER SERVING):

Calories: 250 | Carbs: 8g | Fiber: 2g | Net Carbs: 6g
Protein: 28g | Fats: 12g

Chicken Tikka Masala with Cauliflower Rice

Prep Time: 20 Minutes | **Cook Time:** 30 Minutes |
Serves: 4

INGREDIENTS:

Ingredients for Chicken Tikka Masala:

- ❖ 1 lb chicken breast, cut into bite-sized pieces
- ❖ 1 cup plain Greek yogurt
- ❖ 2 tablespoons tikka masala spice blend
- ❖ 1 tablespoon lemon juice
- ❖ 2 tablespoons olive oil
- ❖ 1 large onion, finely chopped
- ❖ 2 cloves garlic, minced
- ❖ 1 can (14 oz) crushed tomatoes
- ❖ 1/2 cup heavy cream
- ❖ Salt to taste
- ❖ Fresh cilantro for garnish

Ingredients for Cauliflower Rice:

- ❖ 1 large head cauliflower, grated
- ❖ 1 tablespoon olive oil
- ❖ Salt and pepper to taste

INSTRUCTIONS:

1. Marinate the chicken with Greek yogurt, tikka masala spice blend, and lemon juice. Refrigerate for at least 1 hour or overnight.
2. Heat olive oil in a large skillet over medium heat. Add the marinated chicken and cook until browned. Remove chicken and set aside.
3. In the same skillet, add more olive oil if needed, then cook the onion and garlic until softened.
4. Add the crushed tomatoes and bring to a simmer. Return the chicken to the skillet and simmer for 15 minutes.
5. Stir in the heavy cream and cook for an additional 5 minutes. Season with salt to taste.
6. For the cauliflower rice, heat olive oil in a separate skillet. Add the grated cauliflower, salt, and pepper. Cook for 5-7 minutes until tender.
7. Serve the chicken tikka masala over the cauliflower rice, garnished with fresh cilantro.

NUTRITIONAL INFORMATION (PER SERVING):

Calories: 400 | Carbs: 12g | Fiber: 3g | Net Carbs: 9g
Protein: 35g | Fats: 24g

Grilled Chicken and Vegetable Kabobs

Prep Time: 15 Minutes | **Cook Time:** 5 Minutes |
Serves: 4

INGREDIENTS:

- ❖ 1 lb chicken breast, cut into cubes
- ❖ 2 zucchinis, cut into thick slices
- ❖ 2 bell peppers, cut into chunks
- ❖ 1 large red onion, cut into chunks

For the marinade:

- ❖ 1/4 cup olive oil
- ❖ 2 tablespoons lemon juice
- ❖ 2 cloves garlic, minced
- ❖ 1 teaspoon dried oregano
- ❖ Salt and pepper to taste

INSTRUCTIONS:

1. Whisk together all marinade ingredients in a bowl. Add the chicken and vegetables, tossing to coat. Marinate for at least 30 minutes or up to 2 hours in the refrigerator.
2. Preheat the grill to medium-high heat.
3. Thread the marinated chicken and vegetables alternately onto skewers.
4. Grill the kabobs, turning occasionally, until the chicken is cooked through and the vegetables are slightly charred, about 10-15 minutes.
5. Serve hot.

NUTRITIONAL INFORMATION (PER SERVING):

Calories: 300 | Carbs: 10 | Fiber: 2g | Net Carbs: 8g
Protein: 30g | Fats: 16g

Chicken Zoodle Soup

Prep Time: 20 Minutes | **Cook Time:** 30 Minutes |
Serves: 4

INGREDIENTS:

- 1 tablespoon olive oil
- 1/2 onion, chopped
- 2 carrots, sliced
- 2 stalks celery, sliced
- 2 cloves garlic, minced
- Salt and pepper to taste
- 6 cups chicken broth
- 1 lb chicken breast, cooked and shredded
- 2 zucchinis, spiralized into noodles
- Fresh parsley for garnish

INSTRUCTIONS:

1. Heat olive oil in a large pot over medium heat. Add onion, carrots, celery, and garlic. Cook until vegetables are softened, about 5 minutes.
2. Add chicken broth and bring to a boil. Reduce heat and simmer for 15 minutes.
3. Add the cooked, shredded chicken and zucchini noodles to the pot. Cook for an additional 5 minutes, or until the zucchini noodles are tender.
4. Season with salt and pepper to taste.
5. Serve hot, garnished with fresh parsley.

NUTRITIONAL INFORMATION (PER SERVING):

Calories: 220 | Carbs: 8g | Fiber: 2g | Net Carbs: 6g Protein: 30g | Fats: 8g

Thanksgiving Turkey Breast

Prep Time: 20 Minutes | **Cook Time:** 90 Minutes | **Serves:** 6

INGREDIENTS:

- 1 boneless turkey breast (about 3-4 lbs)
- 2 tablespoons olive oil
- 1 tablespoon fresh rosemary, chopped
- 1 tablespoon fresh thyme, chopped
- 2 cloves garlic, minced
- Salt and pepper to taste
- 1/2 cup chicken broth

INSTRUCTIONS:

1. Preheat your oven to 350°F (175°C).
2. In a small bowl, mix together olive oil, rosemary, thyme, garlic, salt, and pepper. Rub this mixture all over the turkey breast.
3. Place the turkey breast in a roasting pan and pour the chicken broth into the bottom of the pan.
4. Roast in the preheated oven for about 1 hour and 30 minutes, or until the internal temperature reaches 165°F (74°C). Baste the turkey occasionally with the pan juices.
5. Let the turkey rest for 10 minutes before slicing and serving.

NUTRITIONAL INFORMATION (PER SERVING):

Calories: 300 | Carbs: 1g | Fiber: 0g | Net Carbs: 1g Protein: 55g | Fats: 7g

Turkey Meatloaf with Sun-Dried Tomatoes

Prep Time: 15 Minutes | **Cook Time:** 1 Hour | **Serves:** 6

INGREDIENTS:

- 2 lbs ground turkey
- 1/2 cup almond flour
- 1/2 cup sun-dried tomatoes, chopped
- 1 onion, finely chopped
- 2 cloves garlic, minced
- 1 egg, beaten
- 2 tablespoons Italian seasoning
- Salt and pepper to taste
- 1/4 cup low-carb ketchup or tomato paste for topping

INSTRUCTIONS:

1. Preheat your oven to 375°F (190°C).
2. In a large bowl, combine ground turkey, almond flour, sun-dried tomatoes, onion, garlic, egg, Italian seasoning, salt, and pepper. Mix until well combined.
3. Shape the mixture into a loaf and place it in a baking dish.
4. Spread the low-carb ketchup or tomato paste over the top of the meatloaf.
5. Bake for 1 hour, or until the meatloaf is cooked through and the top is slightly caramelized.
6. Let the meatloaf rest for 10 minutes before slicing and serving.

NUTRITIONAL INFORMATION (PER SERVING):

Calories: 350 | Carbs: 8g | Fiber: 2g | Net Carbs: 6g
Protein: 40g | Fats: 18g

Chicken Parmesan Stuffed Zucchini Boats

Prep Time: 20 Minutes | **Cook Time:** 25 Minutes | **Serves:** 4

INGREDIENTS:

- 4 medium zucchini, halved lengthwise
- 2 cups cooked and shredded chicken breast
- 1 cup marinara sauce, low-carb
- 1/2 cup grated Parmesan cheese
- 1/2 cup shredded mozzarella cheese
- 1 tablespoon Italian seasoning
- Salt and pepper to taste
- Fresh basil for garnish

INSTRUCTIONS:

1. Preheat your oven to 375°F (190°C).
2. Scoop out the center of each zucchini half to create a "boat."
3. In a bowl, mix the shredded chicken with marinara sauce, Parmesan cheese, Italian seasoning, salt, and pepper.
4. Fill each zucchini boat with the chicken mixture. Top with shredded mozzarella cheese.
5. Place the zucchini boats in a baking dish and bake for 25 minutes, or until the zucchini is tender and the cheese is melted and bubbly.
6. Garnish with fresh basil before serving.

NUTRITIONAL INFORMATION (PER SERVING):

Calories: 250 | Carbs: 10g | Fiber: 3g | Net Carbs: 7g
Protein: 30g | Fats: 10g

Chicken Provençal

Prep Time: 20 Minutes | **Cook Time:** 40 Minutes | **Serves:** 4

INGREDIENTS:

- 4 bone-in, skin-on chicken thighs
- Salt and pepper to taste
- 2 tablespoons olive oil
- 1 onion, sliced
- 3 cloves garlic, minced
- 1 red bell pepper, sliced
- 1 yellow bell pepper, sliced
- 1/2 cup dry white wine (optional, can be replaced with chicken broth)
- 1 can (14 oz) diced tomatoes, drained
- 1 teaspoon herbes de Provence
- 1/4 cup black olives, pitted

INSTRUCTIONS:

1. Preheat your oven to 375°F (190°C).
2. Season chicken thighs with salt and pepper.
3. Heat olive oil in a large oven-proof skillet over medium-high heat. Add the chicken, skin-side down, and cook until the skin is golden and crispy, about 5-7 minutes. Remove chicken and set aside.
4. In the same skillet, add the onion, garlic, and bell peppers. Sauté until softened, about 5 minutes.
5. Add the white wine or chicken broth, scraping up any browned bits from the bottom of the skillet. Simmer until the liquid is reduced by half.
6. Stir in the diced tomatoes and herbes de Provence.
7. Return the chicken to the skillet, nestling it into the vegetables. Scatter the olives around the chicken.
8. Transfer the skillet to the oven and bake for 25-30 minutes, or until the chicken is cooked through.
9. Garnish with fresh parsley before serving.

NUTRITIONAL INFORMATION (PER SERVING):

Calories: 350 | Carbs: 10g | Fiber: 2g | Net Carbs: 8g
Protein: 25g | Fats: 22g

Duck Confit with Cauliflower Mash

Prep Time: 15 Minutes | **Cook Time:** 2 Hours | **Serves:** 4

INGREDIENTS:

Ingredients for Duck Confit:
- 4 duck legs

Ingredients for Cauliflower Mash:
- 1/4 cup heavy cream

- ❖ Salt and pepper to taste
- ❖ 4 cloves garlic, smashed
- ❖ 4 sprigs fresh thyme
- ❖ Duck fat or olive oil, enough to cover the duck legs
- ❖ 1 large head cauliflower, cut into florets
- ❖ 2 tablespoons unsalted butter
- ❖ Salt and pepper to taste

INSTRUCTIONS:

INSTRUCTIONS:

1. For the duck confit, season the duck legs generously with salt and pepper. Place them in a dish with the garlic and thyme, then cover with duck fat or olive oil. Refrigerate overnight.
2. Preheat the oven to 300°F (150°C). Transfer the duck and fat/oil to an oven-proof dish and cover with foil. Bake for 2 hours, or until the meat is tender and easily pulls away from the bone.
3. For the cauliflower mash, steam the cauliflower florets until tender. Blend in a food processor with butter, heavy cream, salt, and pepper until smooth.
4. Serve the duck confit on top of the cauliflower mash.

NUTRITIONAL INFORMATION (PER SERVING):

Calories: 500 | Carbs: 8g | Fiber: 3g | Net Carbs: 5g Protein: 30g | Fats: 38g

Chicken Satay Stir-fry

Prep Time: 20 Minutes | **Cook Time:** 15 Minutes | **Serves:** 4

INGREDIENTS:

- ❖ 1 lb chicken breast, thinly sliced
- ❖ 2 tablespoons coconut oil
- ❖ 1 red bell pepper, sliced
- ❖ 1 yellow bell pepper, sliced
- ❖ 1 zucchini, sliced
- ❖ 1/4 cup peanut butter or almond butter
- ❖ 2 tablespoons soy sauce or tamari
- ❖ 1 tablespoon lime juice
- ❖ 1 teaspoon ginger, grated
- ❖ 1 clove garlic, minced
- ❖ 1/4 cup water
- ❖ Crushed peanuts and fresh cilantro for garnish

INSTRUCTIONS:

1. Heat coconut oil in a large skillet or wok over medium-high heat. Add the chicken and stir-fry until cooked through. Remove and set aside.
2. In the same skillet, add the bell peppers and zucchini. Stir-fry until just tender.
3. In a small bowl, whisk together the peanut or almond butter, soy sauce or tamari, lime juice, ginger, garlic, and water to make the sauce.
4. Return the cooked chicken to the skillet with the vegetables. Pour the sauce over the chicken and vegetables, tossing well to coat everything evenly.
5. Cook for an additional 2-3 minutes, until everything is heated through and the sauce has thickened slightly.
6. Serve hot, garnished with crushed peanuts and fresh cilantro.

NUTRITIONAL INFORMATION (PER SERVING):

Calories: 340 | Carbs: 10g | Fiber: 3g | Net Carbs: 7g Protein: 30g | Fats: 20g

Chapter 7
Fish and Seafood

Lemon Garlic Baked Salmon

Prep Time: 10 Minutes | **Cook Time:** 20 Minutes |
Serves: 4

INGREDIENTS:

- 4 salmon fillets (about 6 ounces each)
- 2 tablespoons olive oil
- 2 cloves garlic, minced
- Juice and zest of 1 lemon
- Salt and pepper to taste
- Fresh dill for garnish

INSTRUCTIONS:

1. Preheat your oven to 400°F (200°C).
2. In a small bowl, mix together the olive oil, minced garlic, lemon juice, and zest. Season with salt and pepper.
3. Place the salmon fillets in a baking dish. Pour the lemon garlic mixture over the salmon, ensuring each fillet is well coated.
4. Bake in the preheated oven for about 15-20 minutes, or until the salmon flakes easily with a fork.
5. Serve the salmon garnished with fresh dill and additional lemon slices if desired.

NUTRITIONAL INFORMATION (PER SERVING):

Calories: 300 | Carbs: 2g | Fiber: 0g | Net Carbs: 2g
Protein: 34g | Fats: 18g

Spicy Shrimp and Avocado Salad

Prep Time: 15 Minutes | **Cook Time:** 5 Minutes |
Serves: 4

INGREDIENTS:

- 1 lb shrimp, peeled and deveined
- 1 tablespoon olive oil
- 1 teaspoon chili powder
- Salt and pepper to taste
- 2 avocados, diced
- 1 cup cherry tomatoes, halved
- 1/4 cup red onion, finely chopped
- Juice of 1 lime
- Fresh cilantro for garnish

INSTRUCTIONS:

1. Heat olive oil in a skillet over medium-high heat. Add shrimp and season with chili powder, salt, and pepper. Cook until shrimp are pink and opaque, about 2-3 minutes per side.
2. In a large bowl, combine the cooked shrimp, diced avocados, cherry tomatoes, and red onion.
3. Drizzle with lime juice and gently toss to combine. Season with additional salt and pepper if needed.
4. Serve the salad garnished with fresh cilantro.

NUTRITIONAL INFORMATION (PER SERVING):

Calories: 280 | Carbs: 10g | Fiber: 6g | Net Carbs: 4g
Protein: 25g | Fats: 18g

Grilled Tilapia with Mango Salsa

Prep Time: 20 Minutes | **Cook Time:** 10 Minutes |
Serves: 4

INGREDIENTS:

Ingredients for Tilapia:

- 4 tilapia fillets
- 2 tablespoons olive oil
- Juice of 1 lime
- 1 teaspoon paprika
- Salt and pepper to taste

Ingredients for Mango Salsa:

- 1 ripe mango, diced
- 1/2 red bell pepper, diced
- 1/4 cup red onion, finely chopped
- 1 jalapeño, seeded and minced (optional)
- Juice of 1 lime
- 2 tablespoons fresh cilantro, chopped
- Salt to taste

INSTRUCTIONS:

1. In a small bowl, whisk together olive oil, lime juice, paprika, salt, and pepper. Marinate the tilapia fillets in this mixture for at least 30 minutes in the refrigerator.
2. Preheat the grill to medium-high heat. Grill the tilapia fillets for about 4-5 minutes on each side, or until the fish flakes easily with a fork.

3. While the fish is grilling, mix together the diced mango, red bell pepper, red onion, jalapeño (if using), lime juice, cilantro, and salt in a bowl to make the mango salsa.
4. Serve the grilled tilapia topped with the mango salsa.

NUTRITIONAL INFORMATION (PER SERVING):

Calories: 250 | Carbs: 12g | Fiber: 2g | Net Carbs: 10g
Protein: 25g | Fats: 12g

Tomato Tuna Melts

Prep Time: 10 Minutes | **Cook Time:** 5 Minutes | **Serves:** 4

INGREDIENTS:

- 4 large tomatoes, halved horizontally
- 2 cans (6 oz each) tuna, drained
- 1/4 cup celery, finely chopped
- 1 tablespoon fresh parsley, chopped
- 1/4 cup mayonnaise
- tablespoons red onion, finely chopped
- Salt and pepper to taste
- 1/2 cup shredded cheddar cheese

INSTRUCTIONS:

1. Preheat a broiler.
2. Scoop out the center of each tomato half to create a small cavity.
3. In a bowl, mix together tuna, mayonnaise, celery, red onion, parsley, salt, and pepper.
4. Fill each tomato half with the tuna mixture.
5. Top each filled tomato with shredded cheddar cheese.
6. Place the tomato halves on a baking sheet and broil for about 5 minutes, or until the cheese is melted and bubbly.
7. Serve immediately.

NUTRITIONAL INFORMATION (PER SERVING):

Calories: 250 | Carbs: 6g | Fiber: 2g | Net Carbs: 4g
Protein: 20g | Fats: 16g

Pan-Seared Scallops with Asparagus

Prep Time: 10 Minutes | **Cook Time:** 10 Minutes | **Serves:** 4

INGREDIENTS:

- 12 large sea scallops, patted dry
- Salt and pepper to taste
- 1 lb asparagus, trimmed and cut into 2-inch pieces
- 2 tablespoons olive oil
- 2 cloves garlic, minced
- 1 tablespoon lemon juice
- 1 tablespoon fresh parsley, chopped

INSTRUCTIONS:

1. Season the scallops with salt and pepper.
2. Heat 1 tablespoon olive oil in a large skillet over high heat. Add the scallops and sear for about 2 minutes on each side, until they have a golden crust. Remove from the skillet and set aside.
3. In the same skillet, add the remaining olive oil and asparagus. Sauté for about 5 minutes until tender but still crisp.
4. Add garlic and cook for another minute until fragrant.
5. Return the scallops to the skillet, add lemon juice, and toss gently to combine.
6. Garnish with fresh parsley and serve immediately.

NUTRITIONAL INFORMATION (PER SERVING):

Calories: 200 | Carbs: 6g | Fiber: 2g | Net Carbs: 4g
Protein: 15g | Fats: 12g

Tuna and Avocado Wraps

Prep Time: 15 Minutes | **Cook Time:** 0 Minute | **Serves:** 4

INGREDIENTS:

- 2 cans (6 oz each) tuna, drained
- 1 ripe avocado, mashed
- 1/4 cup red onion, finely chopped
- 2 tablespoons cilantro, chopped
- Juice of 1 lime
- Salt and pepper to taste

❖ 4 large lettuce leaves (e.g., romaine or butter lettuce)

1. In a bowl, mix together the mashed avocado, tuna, red onion, cilantro, lime juice, salt, and pepper.
2. Lay out the lettuce leaves and divide the tuna mixture among them.
3. Roll up the lettuce leaves to enclose the filling, similar to a wrap.
4. Serve immediately as a light and refreshing meal.

NUTRITIONAL INFORMATION (PER SERVING):

Calories: 180 | Carbs: 5g | Fiber: 3g | Net Carbs: 2g
Protein: 20g | Fats: 10g

Herb-Crusted Cod with Zucchini Noodles

Prep Time: 15 Minutes | **Cook Time:** 15 Minutes |
Serves: 4

INGREDIENTS:

❖ 4 cod fillets (about 6 ounces each)
❖ 2 tablespoons olive oil
❖ 2 tablespoons fresh parsley, finely chopped
❖ 1 teaspoon dried thyme
❖ 1/4 cup almond flour
❖ Salt and pepper to taste
❖ 4 medium zucchinis, spiralized into noodles
❖ 1 tablespoon unsalted butter
❖ 1 clove garlic, minced

INSTRUCTIONS:

1. Preheat your oven to 400°F (200°C). Line a baking sheet with parchment paper.
2. In a shallow dish, combine almond flour, parsley, thyme, salt, and pepper.
3. Brush each cod fillet with olive oil, then press into the herb mixture to coat.
4. Place the coated cod fillets on the prepared baking sheet. Bake for 12-15 minutes, or until the fish flakes easily with a fork.
5. While the fish is baking, heat butter in a large skillet over medium heat. Add garlic and sauté for 1 minute. Add zucchini noodles and cook, stirring frequently, for 2-3 minutes or until just tender.
6. Serve the herb-crusted cod over a bed of zucchini noodles.

NUTRITIONAL INFORMATION (PER SERVING):

Calories: 280 | Carbs: 6g | Fiber: 2g | Net Carbs: 4g
Protein: 30g | Fats: 16g

Lemon Pepper Tilapia with Broccoli and Carrots

Prep Time: 10 Minutes | **Cook Time:** 20 Minutes |
Serves: 4

INGREDIENTS:

❖ 4 tilapia fillets
❖ 2 tablespoons lemon juice
❖ 1 teaspoon black pepper
❖ 1 teaspoon lemon zest
❖ 2 tablespoons olive oil
❖ 2 cups broccoli florets
❖ 1 cup carrot slices
❖ Salt to taste

INSTRUCTIONS:

1. Preheat your oven to 375°F (190°C). Line a baking sheet with foil.
2. In a small bowl, mix lemon juice, lemon zest, and black pepper.
3. Place tilapia fillets on the prepared baking sheet. Drizzle with half the olive oil and the lemon pepper mixture.
4. Toss broccoli and carrots with the remaining olive oil and a pinch of salt. Arrange the vegetables around the fish on the baking sheet.
5. Bake for 18-20 minutes, or until the fish is cooked through and the vegetables are tender.
6. Serve the tilapia with the roasted broccoli and carrots.

NUTRITIONAL INFORMATION (PER SERVING):

Calories: 220 | Carbs: 6g | Fiber: 2g | Net Carbs: 4g
Protein: 25g | Fats: 11g

Shrimp Scampi with Zoodles

Prep Time: 15 Minutes | **Cook Time:** 10 Minutes |
Serves: 4

INGREDIENTS:

- ❖ 1 lb large shrimp, peeled and deveined
- ❖ 3 tablespoons olive oil
- ❖ 3 cloves garlic, minced
- ❖ 1/4 cup white wine (optional, can be replaced with chicken broth)
- ❖ 4 medium zucchinis, spiralized into noodles
- ❖ Juice of 1 lemon
- ❖ 2 tablespoons fresh parsley, chopped
- ❖ Red pepper flakes to taste (optional)
- ❖ Salt and pepper to taste

INSTRUCTIONS:

1. Heat 2 tablespoons of olive oil in a large skillet over medium-high heat. Add garlic and sauté until fragrant, about 1 minute.
2. Add shrimp to the skillet, season with salt and pepper, and cook until they turn pink and opaque, about 2-3 minutes per side. Remove shrimp and set aside.
3. In the same skillet, add the remaining olive oil and zucchini noodles. Sauté for 2-3 minutes or until just tender.
4. Add white wine or chicken broth and lemon juice to the skillet, bringing to a simmer. Cook for 2 minutes, allowing the sauce to reduce slightly.
5. Return the shrimp to the skillet, toss with zoodles and sauce. Heat through.
6. Garnish with fresh parsley and red pepper flakes if desired before serving.

NUTRITIONAL INFORMATION (PER SERVING):

Calories: 250 | Carbs: 8g | Fiber: 2g | Net Carbs: 6g

Protein: 25g | Fats: 12g

Baked Catfish with Olive Tapenade

Prep Time: 15 Minutes | **Cook Time:** 20 Minutes | **Serves:** 4

INGREDIENTS:

For the Olive Tapenade:

- ❖ 1 cup pitted olives (Kalamata or a mix)
- ❖ 4 catfish fillets (about 6 ounces each)
- ❖ Salt and pepper to taste
- ❖ 2 tablespoons capers, rinsed
- ❖ 2 cloves garlic
- ❖ 1 tablespoon lemon juice
- ❖ 3 tablespoons olive oil
- ❖ 1 tablespoon fresh parsley, chopped
- ❖ 2 tablespoons olive oil

INSTRUCTIONS:

1. Preheat your oven to 375°F (190°C).
2. Season the catfish fillets with salt and pepper and drizzle with olive oil. Place them on a baking sheet.
3. Bake in the preheated oven for about 20 minutes, or until the fish flakes easily with a fork.
4. While the fish is baking, make the tapenade by combining olives, capers, garlic, lemon juice, olive oil, and parsley in a food processor. Pulse until the mixture is coarsely chopped.
5. Serve the baked catfish topped with olive tapenade.

NUTRITIONAL INFORMATION (PER SERVING):

Calories: 350 | Carbs: 3g | Fiber: 1g | Net Carbs: 2g

Protein: 25g | Fats: 26g

Crab Stuffed Mushrooms

Prep Time: 20 Minutes | **Cook Time:** 15 Minutes | **Serves:** 4

INGREDIENTS:

- ❖ 16 large mushrooms, stems removed
- ❖ 1 cup crab meat, drained
- ❖ 1/4 cup cream cheese, softened
- ❖ 1 garlic clove, minced
- ❖ 2 tablespoons green onions, finely chopped
- ❖ 1/4 cup grated Parmesan cheese
- ❖ Salt and pepper to taste
- ❖ 1 tablespoon olive oil

INSTRUCTIONS:

1. Preheat your oven to 375°F (190°C).
2. In a bowl, mix together crab meat, cream cheese, green onions, garlic, half of the Parmesan cheese, salt, and pepper.

3. Fill each mushroom cap with the crab mixture and place on a baking sheet.
4. Drizzle the mushrooms with olive oil and sprinkle with the remaining Parmesan cheese.
5. Bake for 15 minutes or until the mushrooms are tender and the tops are golden brown.
6. Serve warm.

NUTRITIONAL INFORMATION (PER SERVING):

Calories: 180 | Carbs: 4g | Fiber: 1g | Net Carbs: 3g
Protein: 12g | Fats: 15g

Mackerel with Mustard Sauce

Prep Time: 10 Minutes | **Cook Time:** 15 Minutes |
Serves: 4

INGREDIENTS:

For the Mackerel:

- 4 mackerel fillets
- Salt and pepper to taste
- 2 tablespoons olive oil

For the Mustard Sauce:

- 2 tablespoons Dijon mustard
- 1 tablespoon olive oil
- 1 tablespoon lemon juice
- 1 teaspoon fresh dill, chopped
- Salt and pepper to taste

INSTRUCTIONS:

1. Season the mackerel fillets with salt and pepper.
2. Heat olive oil in a skillet over medium heat. Add the mackerel fillets, skin-side down, and cook for about 4-5 minutes until the skin is crispy. Flip and cook for another 2-3 minutes until the fish is cooked through.
3. For the mustard sauce, whisk together Dijon mustard, olive oil, lemon juice, dill, salt, and pepper in a bowl until smooth.
4. Serve the mackerel fillets drizzled with the mustard sauce.

NUTRITIONAL INFORMATION (PER SERVING):

Calories: 290 | Carbs: 1g | Fiber: 0g | Net Carbs: 1g
Protein: 23g | Fats: 22g

Grilled Octopus with Lemon and Olive Oil

Prep Time: 20 Minutes | **Cook Time:** 80 Minutes |
Serves: 4

INGREDIENTS:

- 1 whole octopus, cleaned (about 2-3 lbs)
- 1/4 cup olive oil, plus more for grilling
- Juice and zest of 1 lemon
- 2 cloves garlic, minced
- 1 teaspoon dried oregano
- Salt and pepper to taste
- Fresh parsley, chopped for garnish
- Lemon wedges for serving

INSTRUCTIONS:

1. Tenderize the octopus by simmering it in a large pot of salted water for about 1 hour or until tender. Let it cool, then cut into pieces.
2. In a bowl, combine 1/4 cup olive oil, lemon juice and zest, garlic, oregano, salt, and pepper. Add the octopus pieces to the marinade and let sit for at least 30 minutes.
3. Preheat the grill to high heat. Remove the octopus from the marinade and grill for about 3-5 minutes on each side, until charred and crispy.
4. Serve the grilled octopus garnished with fresh parsley and lemon wedges on the side.

NUTRITIONAL INFORMATION (PER SERVING):

Calories: 250 | Carbs: 4g | Fiber: 0g | Net Carbs: 4g
Protein: 35g | Fats: 10g

Baked Cod with Mango Salsa

Prep Time: 15 Minutes | **Cook Time:** 15 Minutes |
Serves: 4

INGREDIENTS:

Ingredients for Mango Salsa:

- 1 ripe mango, diced
- 1/2 red bell pepper, diced
- Juice of 1 lime

Ingredients for Cod:

- 4 cod fillets (about 6 ounces each)
- Salt and pepper to taste
- 2 tablespoons olive oil

- ❖ 1/4 cup red onion, finely chopped
- ❖ 1 jalapeño, seeded and minced (optional)
- ❖ 2 tablespoons fresh cilantro, chopped
- ❖ Salt to taste

INSTRUCTIONS:

1. Preheat your oven to 400°F (200°C).
2. Season the cod fillets with salt and pepper. Place them in a baking dish and drizzle with olive oil.
3. Bake the cod in the preheated oven for about 12-15 minutes, or until the fish flakes easily with a fork.
4. While the cod is baking, combine all the mango salsa ingredients in a bowl and mix well.
5. Serve the baked cod topped with the fresh mango salsa.

NUTRITIONAL INFORMATION (PER SERVING):

Calories: 220 | Carbs: 10g | Fiber: 1g | Net Carbs: 9g

Protein: 25g | Fats: 8g

Clam Chowder with Cauliflower Cream

Prep Time: 15 Minutes | **Cook Time:** 30 Minutes | **Serves:** 4

INGREDIENTS:

- ❖ 1 large head cauliflower, chopped
- ❖ 2 cups vegetable or fish broth
- ❖ 1 cup heavy cream
- ❖ 2 tablespoons butter
- ❖ 2 cloves garlic, minced
- ❖ 1 onion, diced
- ❖ 2 celery stalks, diced
- ❖ 1 lb clams, chopped (canned or fresh)
- ❖ Salt and pepper to taste
- ❖ Fresh thyme for garnish

INSTRUCTIONS:

1. In a large pot, combine the cauliflower and broth. Bring to a boil, then reduce heat and simmer until cauliflower is tender, about 15-20 minutes.
2. Use an immersion blender to puree the cauliflower and broth until smooth. Stir in the heavy cream and set aside.
3. In another pot, melt the butter over medium heat. Add the onion, celery, and garlic, and sauté until softened.
4. Add the clam meat to the pot, and cook for about 5 minutes.
5. Combine the cauliflower cream with the clam mixture. Heat through, but do not boil.
6. Season with salt and pepper to taste.
7. Serve the chowder garnished with fresh thyme.

NUTRITIONAL INFORMATION (PER SERVING):

Calories: 350 | Carbs: 15g | Fiber: 5g | Net Carbs: 10g

Protein: 20g | Fats: 22g

Broiled Lobster Tail with Herb Butter

Prep Time: 10 Minutes | **Cook Time:** 10 Minutes | **Serves:** 4

INGREDIENTS:

- ❖ 4 lobster tails
- ❖ 1/2 cup unsalted butter, softened
- ❖ 1 tablespoon fresh parsley, chopped
- ❖ 1 clove garlic, minced
- ❖ Zest of 1 lemon
- ❖ Salt and pepper to taste

INSTRUCTIONS:

1. Preheat a broiler and position a rack about 6 inches from the heat source.
2. Using kitchen shears, cut the lobster tail shell down the center to the tail fin. Gently pry the shell open and lift the lobster meat out, resting it on top of the shell.
3. In a small bowl, mix together the softened butter, parsley, garlic, lemon zest, salt, and pepper.
4. Spread the herb butter evenly over the lobster meat.
5. Place the lobster tails on a baking sheet and broil for about 8-10 minutes, or until the lobster meat is opaque and the butter is bubbling.
6. Serve immediately, garnished with additional fresh parsley and lemon wedges.

NUTRITIONAL INFORMATION (PER SERVING):

Calories: 250 | Carbs: 1g | Fiber: 0g | Net Carbs: 1g

Protein: 23g | Fats: 18g

Cajun Salmon

Prep Time: 5 Minutes | **Cook Time:** 15 Minutes | **Serves:** 4

INGREDIENTS:

- 4 salmon fillets (about 6 ounces each)
- 2 tablespoons olive oil
- 2 tablespoons Cajun seasoning
- Salt to taste
- Lemon wedges for serving

INSTRUCTIONS:

1. Preheat oven to 400°F (200°C).
2. Rub each salmon fillet with olive oil and coat generously with Cajun seasoning. Season with a little salt if your Cajun seasoning isn't very salty.
3. Place the salmon fillets on a baking sheet lined with parchment paper.
4. Bake in the preheated oven for about 12-15 minutes, or until the salmon flakes easily with a fork.
5. Serve hot with lemon wedges on the side.

NUTRITIONAL INFORMATION (PER SERVING):

Calories: 280 | Carbs: 1g | Fiber: 0g | Net Carbs: 1g
Protein: 35g | Fats: 14g

Sardines with Tomato and Basil

Prep Time: 5 Minutes | **Cook Time:** 5 Minutes | **Serves:** 4

INGREDIENTS:

- 2 cans of sardines in olive oil, drained
- 2 tomatoes, diced
- 1/4 cup fresh basil leaves, chopped
- 2 tablespoons olive oil
- 1 tablespoon balsamic vinegar
- Salt and pepper to taste

INSTRUCTIONS:

1. Heat olive oil in a skillet over medium heat. Add the sardines and cook for 2-3 minutes until warmed through.
2. In a bowl, mix together the diced tomatoes, chopped basil, balsamic vinegar, salt, and pepper.
3. Serve the sardines topped with the tomato and basil mixture.
4. Enjoy as a light entrée or a hearty appetizer.

NUTRITIONAL INFORMATION (PER SERVING):

Calories: 200 | Carbs: 3g | Fiber: 1g | Net Carbs: 2g
Protein: 15g | Fats: 14g

Seafood Paella with Cauliflower Rice

Prep Time: 20 Minutes | **Cook Time:** 30 Minutes | **Serves:** 4

INGREDIENTS:

- 1 large head cauliflower, riced
- 2 tablespoons olive oil
- 1 small onion, diced
- 1 red bell pepper, diced
- 1/2 teaspoon saffron threads
- 1 teaspoon smoked paprika
- Salt and pepper to taste
- 2 cloves garlic, minced
- 1 cup chicken or vegetable broth
- 1/2 lb shrimp, peeled and deveined
- 1/2 lb mussels, cleaned
- 1/2 lb clams, cleaned
- Fresh parsley, chopped for garnish
- Lemon wedges for serving

INSTRUCTIONS:

1. Heat olive oil in a large skillet over medium heat. Add onion, bell pepper, and garlic. Sauté until softened, about 5 minutes.
2. Stir in the riced cauliflower, saffron, smoked paprika, salt, and pepper. Cook for another 5 minutes.
3. Pour in the broth, then arrange the shrimp, mussels, and clams on top of the cauliflower rice. Cover the skillet with a lid and simmer for 15-20 minutes, or until the seafood is cooked and the shellfish have opened. Discard any that do not open.
4. Garnish with fresh parsley and serve with lemon wedges on the side.

NUTRITIONAL INFORMATION (PER SERVING):

Calories: 300 | Carbs: 12g | Fiber: 3g | Net Carbs: 9g
Protein: 25g | Fats: 16g

Caribbean Haddock in a Packet

Prep Time: 15 Minutes | **Cook Time:** 20 Minutes | **Serves:** 4

INGREDIENTS:

- 4 haddock fillets (about 6 ounces each)
- 2 tablespoons olive oil
- 1 lime, sliced
- 1 mango, diced
- 1 red bell pepper, thinly sliced
- 1 small red onion, thinly sliced
- 1 jalapeño, seeded and minced (optional)
- Salt and pepper to taste
- Fresh cilantro for garnish

INSTRUCTIONS:

1. Preheat your oven to 400°F (200°C).
2. Cut 4 large pieces of parchment paper or aluminum foil. Place a haddock fillet on each piece.
3. Drizzle each fillet with olive oil and season with salt and pepper. Top with lime slices, diced mango, bell pepper slices, onion slices, and minced jalapeño if using.
4. Fold the parchment paper or foil over the fish and vegetables, sealing the edges to create a packet.
5. Bake for 20 minutes or until the fish is cooked through and flakes easily.
6. Carefully open the packets (watch for steam) and garnish with fresh cilantro before serving.

NUTRITIONAL INFORMATION (PER SERVING):

Calories: 260 | Carbs: 12g | Fiber: 2g | Net Carbs: 10g
Protein: 35g | Fats: 8g

Roasted Red Snapper and Shrimp in Parchment

Prep Time: 20 Minutes | **Cook Time:** 25 Minutes | **Serves:** 4

INGREDIENTS:

- 4 red snapper fillets (about 6 ounces each)
- 12 large shrimp, peeled and deveined
- 4 sprigs fresh thyme
- 4 tablespoons olive oil
- 2 tomatoes, thinly sliced
- Lemon slices for garnish
- 2 zucchinis, thinly sliced
- Salt and pepper to taste

INSTRUCTIONS:

1. Preheat your oven to 400°F (200°C).
2. Cut 4 large pieces of parchment paper. Place a snapper fillet and 3 shrimp on each piece.
3. Drizzle each with 1 tablespoon of olive oil and season with salt and pepper. Arrange tomato and zucchini slices over the fish and shrimp. Top each with a sprig of thyme.
4. Fold the parchment paper over the ingredients, sealing the edges to create a packet.
5. Bake for 25 minutes or until the fish is cooked through and the shrimp are pink and opaque.
6. Carefully open the packets and serve with lemon slices for garnish.

NUTRITIONAL INFORMATION (PER SERVING):

Calories: 360 | Carbs: 6g | Fiber: 2g | Net Carbs: 4g
Protein: 40g | Fats: 16g

Baked Halibut with Capers and Olives

Prep Time: 10 Minutes | **Cook Time:** 15 Minutes | **Serves:** 4

INGREDIENTS:

- 4 halibut fillets (about 6 ounces each)
- 2 tablespoons olive oil
- Salt and pepper to taste
- 1/4 cup capers, drained
- 1/4 cup olives, pitted and sliced
- 2 cloves garlic, minced
- 1 lemon, sliced
- Fresh parsley, chopped for garnish

INSTRUCTIONS:

1. Preheat your oven to 400°F (200°C).
2. Place halibut fillets in a baking dish. Drizzle with olive oil and season with salt and pepper.
3. Scatter capers, olives, and minced garlic around the fish. Top each fillet with lemon slices.
4. Bake in the preheated oven for about 15 minutes, or

until the fish flakes easily with a fork.
5. Garnish with fresh parsley before serving.

Calories: 220 | Carbs: 2g | Fiber: 0.5g | Net Carbs: 1.5g
Protein: 25g | Fats: 12g

Baked Oysters

Prep Time: 15 Minutes | **Cook Time:** 10 Minutes |
Serves: 4

INGREDIENTS:

- 12 fresh oysters, shucked
- 1/4 cup grated Parmesan cheese
- 1/4 cup unsalted butter, softened
- 2 cloves garlic, minced
- 1 tablespoon fresh parsley, chopped
- 1 teaspoon lemon zest
- Salt and pepper to taste
- Lemon wedges for serving

INSTRUCTIONS:

1. Preheat your oven to 425°F (220°C).
2. Arrange the shucked oysters on a baking sheet.
3. In a small bowl, mix together the Parmesan cheese, softened butter, minced garlic, parsley, and lemon zest. Season with salt and pepper.
4. Place a dollop of the cheese and butter mixture on top of each oyster.
5. Bake in the preheated oven for about 10 minutes, or until the topping is golden and bubbly.
6. Serve hot with lemon wedges on the side.

NUTRITIONAL INFORMATION (PER SERVING):

Calories: 180 | Carbs: 2g | Fiber: 0g | Net Carbs: 2g
Protein: 6g | Fats: 16g

Seared Tuna Salad with Avocado

Prep Time: 15 Minutes | **Cook Time:** 5 Minutes |
Serves: 4

INGREDIENTS:

- 4 tuna steaks (about 6 ounces each)
- Salt and pepper to taste
- 2 tablespoons olive oil
- 4 cups mixed salad greens
- 1 avocado, sliced

For the dressing:

- 3 tablespoons olive oil
- 1 tablespoon balsamic vinegar
- 1 teaspoon Dijon mustard
- Salt and pepper to taste

INSTRUCTIONS:

1. Season the tuna steaks with salt and pepper.
2. Heat olive oil in a skillet over high heat. Sear the tuna for about 2 minutes on each side (for medium-rare), or until cooked to your liking.
3. In a large bowl, toss the mixed salad greens and avocado slices.
4. Whisk together the ingredients for the dressing in a small bowl.
5. Slice the seared tuna and arrange on top of the salad.
6. Drizzle the dressing over the salad and serve immediately.

NUTRITIONAL INFORMATION (PER SERVING):

Calories: 350 | Carbs: 6g | Fiber: 4g | Net Carbs: 2g
Protein: 30g | Fats: 22g

Sea Bass with Ginger Sauce

Prep Time: 15 Minutes | **Cook Time:** 20 Minutes |
Serves: 4

INGREDIENTS:

- 4 sea bass fillets (about 6 ounces each)
- Salt and pepper to taste
- 2 tablespoons olive oil
- 1 tablespoon fresh ginger, grated
- 1/4 cup soy sauce (or tamari for a gluten-free option)
- 2 cloves garlic, minced
- 1 tablespoon sesame oil
- 1 teaspoon honey (optional, can omit for lower carbs)
- 2 green onions, thinly sliced
- 1 tablespoon sesame seeds

INSTRUCTIONS:

1. Preheat oven to 375°F (190°C).
2. Season the sea bass fillets with salt and pepper.
3. Heat olive oil in a skillet over medium-high heat. Sear the fillets for about 2 minutes on each side until golden brown.
4. Transfer the fillets to a baking dish.
5. In the same skillet, add ginger and garlic, and sauté for about 1 minute until fragrant.
6. Stir in soy sauce (or tamari), sesame oil, and honey. Simmer for 2-3 minutes to combine flavors.
7. Pour the ginger sauce over the sea bass fillets.
8. Bake in the preheated oven for 12-15 minutes, or until the fish flakes easily with a fork.
9. Garnish with green onions and sesame seeds before serving.

NUTRITIONAL INFORMATION (PER SERVING):

Calories: 300 | Carbs: 3g | Fiber: 0.5g | Net Carbs: 2.5g
Protein: 30g | Fats: 18g

Blackened Pollock

Prep Time: 10 Minutes | **Cook Time:** 10 Minutes | **Serves:** 4

INGREDIENTS:

* 4 pollock fillets (about 6 ounces each)
* 2 tablespoons olive oil
* 1 tablespoon paprika
* 1 teaspoon garlic powder
* 1 teaspoon onion powder
* 1/2 teaspoon cayenne pepper (adjust to taste)
* 1/2 teaspoon dried thyme
* 1/2 teaspoon dried oregano
* Salt and pepper to taste

INSTRUCTIONS:

1. In a small bowl, mix together paprika, garlic powder, onion powder, cayenne pepper, thyme, oregano, salt, and pepper to create the blackening seasoning.
2. Rub the seasoning mixture generously onto both sides of each pollock fillet.
3. Heat olive oil in a large skillet over medium-high heat.
4. Place the seasoned fillets in the skillet and cook for about 4-5 minutes on each side, until the seasoning is blackened and the fish is cooked through.
5. Serve immediately.

NUTRITIONAL INFORMATION (PER SERVING):

Calories: 200 | Carbs: 2g | Fiber: 1g | Net Carbs: 1g
Protein: 25g | Fats: 10g

Cajun Catfish with Collard Greens

Prep Time: 15 Minutes | **Cook Time:** 30 Minutes | **Serves:** 4

INGREDIENTS:

Ingredients for Cajun Catfish:

* 4 catfish fillets (about 6 ounces each)
* 2 tablespoons Cajun seasoning
* 1 tablespoon olive oil

Ingredients for Collard Greens:

* 1 lb collard greens, stems removed and chopped
* 1 tablespoon olive oil
* 2 cloves garlic, minced
* 1/2 cup chicken broth
* Salt and pepper to taste
* 1 tablespoon apple cider vinegar

INSTRUCTIONS:

1. Season the catfish fillets on both sides with Cajun seasoning.
2. Heat olive oil in a skillet over medium-high heat. Add the catfish and cook for about 4-5 minutes on each side, until cooked through and slightly crispy on the outside.
3. For the collard greens, heat olive oil in a large pot over medium heat. Add garlic and sauté until fragrant.
4. Add the chopped collard greens and chicken broth. Cover and cook for about 20 minutes, or until the greens are tender.
5. Season with salt, pepper, and apple cider vinegar.
6. Serve the Cajun catfish with a side of collard greens.

NUTRITIONAL INFORMATION (PER SERVING):

Calories: 300 | Carbs: 5g | Fiber: 3g | Net Carbs: 2g
Protein: 25g | Fats: 18g

Salmon Patties with Dill Sauce

Prep Time: 20 Minutes | **Cook Time:** 10 Minutes |
Serves: 3

INGREDIENTS:

Ingredients for Salmon Patties:

- 2 cans (6 oz each) wild-caught salmon, drained and flaked
- 1/4 cup almond flour
- 2 green onions, finely chopped
- 1 egg, beaten
- 1 tablespoon fresh dill, chopped
- Salt and pepper to taste
- 2 tablespoons olive oil for frying

Ingredients for Dill Sauce:

- 1/2 cup Greek yogurt
- 1 tablespoon fresh dill, chopped
- 1 teaspoon lemon juice
- Salt and pepper to

INSTRUCTIONS:

1. In a large bowl, mix together the salmon, almond flour, green onions, egg, dill, salt, and pepper until well combined.
2. Form the mixture into 8 patties.
3. Heat olive oil in a large skillet over medium heat. Fry the patties for about 4-5 minutes on each side, until golden and crispy.
4. For the dill sauce, mix together Greek yogurt, dill, lemon juice, salt, and pepper in a small bowl.
5. Serve the salmon patties with the dill sauce on the side.

NUTRITIONAL INFORMATION (PER SERVING):

Calories: 280 | Carbs: 3g | Fiber: 1g | Net Carbs: 2g
Protein: 25g | Fats: 18g

Grilled Swordfish with Eggplant Caponata

Prep Time: 30 Minutes | **Cook Time:** 20 Minutes |
Serves: 4

INGREDIENTS:

Ingredients for Swordfish:

Ingredients for Eggplant Caponata:

- 4 swordfish steaks (about 6 ounces each)
- Salt and pepper to taste
- 2 tablespoons olive oil

- 1 large eggplant, diced
- 2 tablespoons olive oil
- 1 onion, diced
- 2 cloves garlic, minced
- 1 bell pepper, diced
- 1 can (14 oz) diced tomatoes, drained
- 2 tablespoons capers
- 1/4 cup olives, chopped
- 2 tablespoons balsamic vinegar
- Salt and pepper to taste

INSTRUCTIONS:

1. Preheat your grill to medium-high heat.
2. Season swordfish steaks with salt and pepper and drizzle with olive oil. Grill for about 4-5 minutes on each side, until cooked through.
3. For the caponata, heat olive oil in a large skillet over medium heat. Add eggplant and cook until it begins to soften. Add onion, garlic, and bell pepper, cooking until softened.
4. Stir in diced tomatoes, capers, olives, and balsamic vinegar. Simmer for about 10 minutes until the vegetables are tender and the flavors meld. Season with salt and pepper.
5. Serve the grilled swordfish topped with eggplant caponata and garnished with fresh basil.

NUTRITIONAL INFORMATION (PER SERVING):

Calories: 400 | Carbs: 15g | Fiber: 5g | Net Carbs: 10g
Protein: 35g | Fats: 22g

Shrimp Creole

Prep Time: 15 Minutes | **Cook Time:** 30 Minutes |
Serves: 4

INGREDIENTS:

- 1 lb large shrimp, peeled and deveined
- 2 tablespoons olive oil
- 1 onion, diced
- 1 bell pepper, diced
- 2 celery stalks, diced
- 2 cloves garlic, minced
- 1 teaspoon paprika

* 1 can (14 oz) diced tomatoes
* 2 tablespoons fresh parsley, chopped
* Salt and pepper to taste
* 1/2 teaspoon cayenne pepper (adjust to taste)
* 1 green onion, thinly sliced for garnish

INSTRUCTIONS:

1. Heat olive oil in a large skillet over medium heat. Add onion, bell pepper, celery, and garlic. Sauté until vegetables are softened, about 5 minutes.
2. Stir in diced tomatoes, paprika, cayenne pepper, salt, and pepper. Bring to a simmer and cook for about 20 minutes, until the sauce thickens slightly.
3. Add the shrimp to the skillet, stirring into the sauce. Cook for about 5 minutes, or until the shrimp are pink and cooked through.
4. Stir in fresh parsley and adjust seasoning if necessary.
5. Serve the shrimp creole garnished with green onion slices.

NUTRITIONAL INFORMATION (PER SERVING):

Calories: 250 | Carbs: 10g | Fiber: 3g | Net Carbs: 7g
Protein: 25g | Fats: 12g

Flounder Roll-Ups with Spinach and Feta

Prep Time: 20 Minutes | **Cook Time:** 25 Minutes | **Serves:** 4

INGREDIENTS:

* 4 flounder fillets (about 6 ounces each)
* Salt and pepper to taste
* 1/2 cup feta cheese, crumbled
* 1 tablespoon olive oil
* 2 cups fresh spinach, chopped
* 1/2 teaspoon garlic powder
* 1 lemon, sliced for garnish

INSTRUCTIONS:

1. Preheat oven to 350°F (175°C).
2. Season the flounder fillets with salt, pepper, and garlic powder.
3. Lay each fillet flat and distribute the spinach and feta cheese evenly among them.
4. Carefully roll up each fillet and secure with a toothpick.
5. Place the roll-ups in a baking dish and drizzle with olive oil.
6. Bake in the preheated oven for about 20-25 minutes, or until the fish flakes easily with a fork.
7. Serve the flounder roll-ups garnished with lemon slices.

NUTRITIONAL INFORMATION (PER SERVING):

Calories: 220 | Carbs: 2g | Fiber: 1g | Net Carbs: 1g
Protein: 30g | Fats: 10g

Prawn Curry with Coconut Milk

Prep Time: 15 Minutes | **Cook Time:** 20 Minutes | **Serves:** 4

INGREDIENTS:

* 1 lb prawns, peeled and deveined
* 1 tablespoon olive oil
* 1 tablespoon curry powder
* 2 cloves garlic, minced
* 1 teaspoon ginger, grated
* 1 onion, chopped
* 1 can (14 oz) coconut milk
* 1/2 cup diced tomatoes
* Salt to taste
* Fresh cilantro for garnish

INSTRUCTIONS:

1. Heat olive oil in a large skillet over medium heat. Add the onion, garlic, and ginger, and sauté until softened.
2. Stir in the curry powder and cook for another minute until fragrant.
3. Pour in the coconut milk and diced tomatoes. Bring to a simmer and cook for about 5 minutes.
4. Add the prawns to the skillet and cook until they are pink and cooked through, about 5-7 minutes.
5. Season with salt to taste.
6. Serve the prawn curry garnished with fresh cilantro.

NUTRITIONAL INFORMATION (PER SERVING):

Calories: 300 | Carbs: 6g | Fiber: 1g | Net Carbs: 5g
Protein: 25g | Fats: 20g

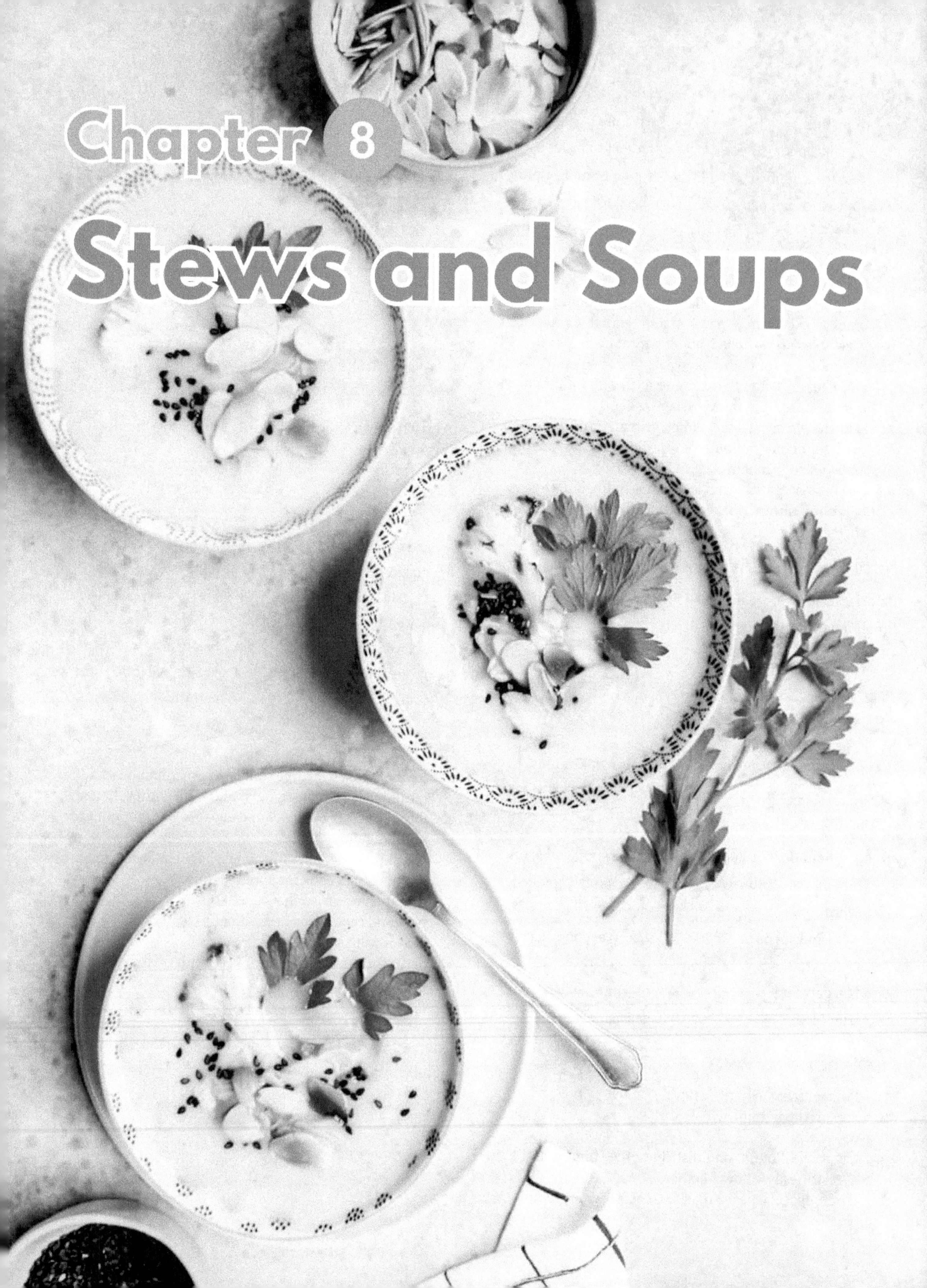

Chapter 8
Stews and Soups

Prep Time: 20 Minutes | **Cook Time:** 90 Minutes |
Serves: 4

INGREDIENTS:

- 1 lb beef stew meat, cut into 1-inch cubes
- 2 tablespoons olive oil
- 1 onion, chopped
- 2 cloves garlic, minced
- 1 lb mushrooms, sliced
- 2 carrots, chopped
- 2 stalks celery, chopped
- 4 cups beef broth
- 1 teaspoon thyme
- Salt and pepper to taste
- 2 tablespoons fresh parsley, chopped for garnish

INSTRUCTIONS:

1. Heat 1 tablespoon olive oil in a large pot over medium-high heat. Add the beef cubes and brown on all sides. Remove beef and set aside.
2. In the same pot, add the remaining olive oil, onion, and garlic. Sauté until translucent.
3. Add mushrooms, carrots, and celery to the pot and cook until they start to soften.
4. Return the beef to the pot. Add beef broth and thyme. Season with salt and pepper.
5. Bring to a boil, then reduce heat to low. Cover and simmer for 1 hour 30 minutes, or until the beef is tender.
6. Garnish with fresh parsley before serving.

NUTRITIONAL INFORMATION (PER SERVING):

Calories: 350 | Carbs: 10g | Fiber: 2g | Net Carbs: 8g
Protein: 35g | Fats: 18g

Cream of Asparagus Soup

Prep Time: 10 Minutes | **Cook Time:** 30 Minutes |
Serves: 4

INGREDIENTS:

- 2 lbs asparagus, trimmed and chopped
- 1 tablespoon olive oil
- 1 onion, chopped
- 1/2 cup heavy cream
- 2 cloves garlic, minced
- 4 cups vegetable broth
- Salt and pepper to taste
- Fresh chives, chopped for garnish

INSTRUCTIONS:

1. Heat olive oil in a large pot over medium heat. Add onion and garlic, sautéing until soft.
2. Add asparagus and cook for 5 minutes, stirring occasionally.
3. Pour in vegetable broth and bring to a boil. Reduce heat and simmer for 20 minutes, or until asparagus is very tender.
4. Use an immersion blender to puree the soup until smooth.
5. Stir in heavy cream and season with salt and pepper. Heat through.
6. Serve garnished with fresh chives.

NUTRITIONAL INFORMATION (PER SERVING):

Calories: 200 | Carbs: 12g | Fiber: 4g | Net Carbs: 8g
Protein: 6g | Fats: 14g

Chicken and Vegetable Soup

Prep Time: 15 Minutes | **Cook Time:** 40 Minutes |
Serves: 4

INGREDIENTS:

- 1 lb chicken breast, diced
- 2 tablespoons olive oil
- 1 onion, chopped
- 2 carrots, chopped
- 2 stalks celery, chopped
- 2 cloves garlic, minced
- 6 cups chicken broth
- 1 cup broccoli florets
- 1 cup cauliflower florets
- Salt and pepper to taste
- Fresh parsley, chopped for garnish

INSTRUCTIONS:

1. Heat olive oil in a large pot over medium heat. Add chicken and cook until browned. Remove chicken and set aside.
2. In the same pot, add onion, carrots, celery, and garlic. Cook until vegetables are soft.
3. Return the chicken to the pot. Add chicken broth and bring to a boil.
4. Reduce heat and add broccoli and cauliflower. Simmer

for 20 minutes, or until vegetables are tender and chicken is cooked through.
5. Season with salt and pepper.
6. Serve garnished with fresh parsley.

NUTRITIONAL INFORMATION (PER SERVING):

Calories: 250 | Carbs: 10g | Fiber: 3g | Net Carbs: 7g
Protein: 30g | Fats: 10g

Spicy Tomato and Seafood Stew

Prep Time: 15 Minutes | **Cook Time:** 30 Minutes |
Serves: 4

INGREDIENTS:

- 1 tablespoon olive oil
- 1 onion, chopped
- 2 cloves garlic, minced
- 1 red chili pepper, seeded and finely chopped (adjust to taste)
- 1 can (14 oz) diced tomatoes
- 2 cups fish or vegetable broth
- 1/2 lb shrimp, peeled and deveined
- 1/2 lb scallops
- 1/2 lb firm white fish (like cod), cut into chunks
- Salt and pepper to taste

INSTRUCTIONS:

1. Heat olive oil in a large pot over medium heat. Add onion, garlic, and chili pepper. Sauté until onion is translucent.
2. Stir in diced tomatoes and broth. Bring to a simmer and cook for 15 minutes.
3. Add shrimp, scallops, and white fish to the pot. Season with salt and pepper. Simmer for 10-15 minutes, or until seafood is cooked through.
4. Garnish with fresh parsley before serving.

NUTRITIONAL INFORMATION (PER SERVING):

Calories: 250 | Carbs: 8g | Fiber: 2g | Net Carbs: 6g
Protein: 35g | Fats: 8g

Pumpkin and Chicken Stew

Prep Time: 20 Minutes | **Cook Time:** 40 Minutes |
Serves: 4

INGREDIENTS:

- 1 lb chicken breast, cut into chunks
- 2 tablespoons olive oil
- 1 onion, chopped
- 2 cloves garlic, minced
- 2 cups pumpkin, peeled and cubed
- 4 cups chicken broth
- 1 teaspoon ground cumin
- 1/2 teaspoon ground cinnamon
- Salt and pepper to taste
- Fresh cilantro, chopped for garnish

INSTRUCTIONS:

1. Heat olive oil in a large pot over medium heat. Add chicken chunks and brown on all sides. Remove chicken and set aside.
2. In the same pot, add onion and garlic. Sauté until soft.
3. Add pumpkin, chicken broth, cumin, and cinnamon to the pot. Bring to a simmer and cook for 20 minutes, or until pumpkin is tender.
4. Return chicken to the pot and cook for an additional 10-15 minutes, until chicken is cooked through.
5. Season with salt and pepper to taste.
6. Serve garnished with fresh cilantro.

NUTRITIONAL INFORMATION (PER SERVING):

Calories: 300 | Carbs: 10g | Fiber: 2g | Net Carbs: 8g
Protein: 30g | Fats: 14g

Italian Sausage and Kale Soup

Prep Time: 15 Minutes | **Cook Time:** 30 Minutes |
Serves: 4

INGREDIENTS:

- 1 lb Italian sausage, casing removed
- 1 tablespoon olive oil
- 1 onion, chopped
- 2 cloves garlic, minced
- 4 cups chicken broth
- 2 cups kale, chopped
- 1 cup heavy cream
- Salt and pepper to taste
- Grated Parmesan cheese for garnish

1. In a large pot, cook Italian sausage over medium heat until browned, breaking it apart with a spoon. Remove sausage and set aside.
2. In the same pot, add olive oil, onion, and garlic. Sauté until onion is soft.
3. Add chicken broth and bring to a simmer. Add kale and cook until tender, about 10 minutes.
4. Return sausage to the pot. Stir in heavy cream and heat through without boiling.
5. Season with salt and pepper to taste.
6. Serve garnished with grated Parmesan cheese.

NUTRITIONAL INFORMATION (PER SERVING):

Calories: 450 | Carbs: 8g | Fiber: 1g | Net Carbs: 7g
Protein: 18g | Fats: 38g

Broccoli Cheddar Soup

Prep Time: 10 Minutes | **Cook Time:** 20 Minutes |
Serves: 4

INGREDIENTS:

- 4 cups broccoli florets, chopped
- 1 tablespoon olive oil
- 1 small onion, diced
- 2 cloves garlic, minced
- 3 cups chicken or vegetable broth
- 1 cup heavy cream
- 1 1/2 cups shredded cheddar cheese
- Salt and pepper to taste

INSTRUCTIONS:

1. Heat olive oil in a large pot over medium heat. Add onion and garlic, and sauté until translucent.
2. Add broccoli florets and broth to the pot. Bring to a boil, then reduce heat and simmer until broccoli is tender, about 10 minutes.
3. Use an immersion blender to partially blend the soup, leaving some broccoli chunks for texture.
4. Stir in the heavy cream and bring the soup back to a simmer.
5. Gradually add shredded cheddar cheese, stirring until melted and smooth. Season with salt and pepper.
6. Serve the soup hot.

NUTRITIONAL INFORMATION (PER SERVING):

Calories: 400 | Carbs: 8g | Fiber: 2g | Net Carbs: 6g
Protein: 16g | Fats: 34g

Cauli-Curry Bean Soup

Prep Time: 15 Minutes | **Cook Time:** 25 Minutes |
Serves: 4

INGREDIENTS:

- 1 large cauliflower, cut into florets
- 1 tablespoon olive oil
- 1 tablespoon curry powder
- 1 can (14 oz) coconut milk
- 4 cups vegetable broth
- 1 onion, chopped
- 1 can (14 oz) white beans, drained and rinsed
- Salt and pepper to taste
- Fresh cilantro for garnish

INSTRUCTIONS:

1. In a large pot, heat olive oil over medium heat. Add onion and curry powder, cooking until onion is soft and fragrant.
2. Add cauliflower florets and vegetable broth to the pot. Bring to a boil, then reduce heat and simmer until cauliflower is tender, about 15 minutes.
3. Stir in coconut milk and white beans. Continue to simmer for an additional 10 minutes.
4. Use an immersion blender to blend the soup to your desired consistency.
5. Season with salt and pepper to taste.
6. Serve garnished with fresh cilantro.

NUTRITIONAL INFORMATION (PER SERVING):

Calories: 300 | Carbs: 22g | Fiber: 7g | Net Carbs: 15g
Protein: 10g | Fats: 20g

Egg Drop Soup with Spinach

Prep Time: 5 Minutes | **Cook Time:** 10 Minutes |
Serves: 4

INGREDIENTS:

- 4 cups chicken broth
- 2 eggs, beaten

❖ 1 cup baby spinach, chopped
❖ 1 teaspoon sesame oil
❖ Salt and white pepper to taste
❖ Green onions, chopped for garnish

INSTRUCTIONS:

1. Bring the chicken broth to a simmer in a large pot over medium heat.
2. Slowly pour the beaten eggs into the simmering broth, stirring gently with a fork to form thin strands of egg.
3. Add chopped spinach to the pot and cook until just wilted, about 1 minute.
4. Stir in sesame oil and season with salt and white pepper to taste.
5. Serve the soup hot, garnished with chopped green onions.

NUTRITIONAL INFORMATION (PER SERVING):

Calories: 80 | Carbs: 1g | Fiber: 0g | Net Carbs: 1g Protein: 6g | Fats: 5g

Fresh Fish Chowder

Prep Time: 15 Minutes | **Cook Time:** 30 Minutes | **Serves:** 4

INGREDIENTS:

❖ 1 lb fresh white fish fillets (e.g., cod, haddock), cut into chunks
❖ 2 tablespoons olive oil
❖ 1 onion, diced
❖ 2 cloves garlic, minced
❖ 2 cups cauliflower florets, chopped into small pieces
❖ 3 cups fish or vegetable broth
❖ 1 cup heavy cream
❖ Salt and pepper to taste
❖ Fresh parsley, chopped for garnish

INSTRUCTIONS:

1. Heat olive oil in a large pot over medium heat. Add onion and garlic, and sauté until softened.
2. Add cauliflower florets and broth to the pot. Bring to a simmer and cook until the cauliflower is tender, about 15 minutes.
3. Use an immersion blender to blend the mixture until smooth to create a creamy base.

4. Add the fish chunks to the pot. Simmer gently for about 10 minutes, or until the fish is cooked through and flakes easily.
5. Stir in the heavy cream and heat through without boiling. Season with salt and pepper.
6. Serve the chowder hot, garnished with fresh parsley.

NUTRITIONAL INFORMATION (PER SERVING):

Calories: 350 | Carbs: 8g | Fiber: 2g | Net Carbs: 6g Protein: 25g | Fats: 4g

Turkey Chili with Beans

Prep Time: 15 Minutes | **Cook Time:** 45 Minutes | **Serves:** 4

INGREDIENTS:

❖ 1 lb ground turkey
❖ 1 tablespoon olive oil
❖ 1 onion, diced
❖ 2 tablespoons chili powder
❖ 1 can (14 oz) diced tomatoes
❖ 1 can (14 oz) low-carb beans (e.g., black soybeans)
❖ 2 cloves garlic, minced
❖ 1 teaspoon ground cumin
❖ Salt and pepper to taste
❖ Fresh cilantro, chopped for garnish
❖ Shredded cheddar cheese for garnish (optional)

INSTRUCTIONS:

1. Heat olive oil in a large pot over medium heat. Add the ground turkey, onion, and garlic. Cook until the turkey is browned and the onion is soft.
2. Stir in diced tomatoes (with juice), beans, chili powder, and cumin. Season with salt and pepper.
3. Bring to a boil, then reduce heat and simmer uncovered for about 30 minutes, stirring occasionally.
4. Serve the chili garnished with fresh cilantro and shredded cheddar cheese if desired.

NUTRITIONAL INFORMATION (PER SERVING):

Calories: 300 | Carbs: 10g | Fiber: 2g | Net Carbs: 8g Protein: 30g | Fats: 14g

Creamy Cauliflower and Leek Soup

Prep Time: 10 Minutes | **Cook Time:** 25 Minutes | **Serves:** 4

INGREDIENTS:

- 1 large cauliflower, cut into florets
- 2 leeks, white and light green parts only, cleaned and sliced
- 2 tablespoons olive oil
- 4 cups vegetable broth
- 1 cup heavy cream
- Salt and pepper to taste
- Fresh chives, chopped for garnish

INSTRUCTIONS:

1. Heat olive oil in a large pot over medium heat. Add leeks and sauté until softened, about 5 minutes.
2. Add cauliflower florets and vegetable broth. Bring to a boil, then reduce heat and simmer until cauliflower is very tender, about 15 minutes.
3. Use an immersion blender to blend the soup until smooth.
4. Stir in the heavy cream and heat through. Season with salt and pepper.
5. Serve the soup hot, garnished with fresh chives.

NUTRITIONAL INFORMATION (PER SERVING):

Calories: 280 | Carbs: 12g | Fiber: 3g | Net Carbs: 9g
Protein: 5g | Fats: 24g

Hungarian Goulash

Prep Time: 20 Minutes | **Cook Time:** 90 Minutes | **Serves:** 4

INGREDIENTS:

- 1 lb beef stew meat, cut into 1-inch cubes
- 2 tablespoons olive oil
- 1 large onion, chopped
- 2 cups beef broth
- 2 cloves garlic, minced
- 2 tablespoons paprika (preferably Hungarian)
- 1 teaspoon caraway seeds
- 1 can (14 oz) diced tomatoes, undrained
- 1 red bell pepper, chopped
- 1 green bell pepper, chopped
- Salt and pepper to taste
- Sour cream for garnish (optional)

INSTRUCTIONS:

1. Start by heating olive oil in a large pot over medium-high heat. Add beef cubes and brown on all sides. Remove beef and set aside.
2. In the same pot, add onion and garlic, cooking until softened.
3. Return beef to the pot, along with paprika and caraway seeds. Stir well to coat the beef.
4. Add diced tomatoes and beef broth. Bring to a boil, then reduce heat, cover, and simmer for 1 hour.
5. Add chopped bell peppers and continue to simmer, uncovered, for an additional 30 minutes, or until beef is tender and sauce has thickened.
6. Season with salt and pepper to taste.
7. Serve hot, garnished with a dollop of sour cream if desired.

NUTRITIONAL INFORMATION (PER SERVING):

Calories: 350 | Carbs: 10g | Fiber: 3g | Net Carbs: 7g
Protein: 35g | Fats: 18g

Minestrone with Zucchini Noodles

Prep Time: 15 Minutes | **Cook Time:** 30 Minutes | **Serves:** 4

INGREDIENTS:

- 2 tablespoons olive oil
- 1 onion, diced
- 2 carrots, diced
- 2 stalks celery, diced
- 2 cloves garlic, minced
- 1 can (14 oz) diced tomatoes
- 1 teaspoon dried Italian herbs
- 4 cups vegetable broth
- 2 zucchinis, spiralized into noodles
- 1 can (14 oz) white beans, drained and rinsed
- Salt and pepper to taste
- Fresh basil for garnish

INSTRUCTIONS:

1. Heat olive oil in a large pot over medium heat. Add

onion, carrots, celery, and garlic, cooking until vegetables are softened.

2. Stir in diced tomatoes (with juice), vegetable broth, and Italian herbs. Bring to a boil, then reduce heat and simmer for about 20 minutes.
3. Add zucchini noodles and white beans to the pot. Cook for an additional 5-10 minutes, or until zucchini noodles are tender.
4. Season with salt and pepper to taste.
5. Serve hot, garnished with fresh basil.

NUTRITIONAL INFORMATION (PER SERVING):

Calories: 250 | Carbs: 30g | Fiber: 8g | Net Carbs: 22g
Protein: 10g | Fats: 10g

Chicken Brunswick Stew

Prep Time: 20 Minutes | **Cook Time:** 1 Hour | **Serves:** 4

INGREDIENTS:

- 1 lb chicken breast, cooked and shredded
- 2 tablespoons olive oil
- 1 onion, diced
- 2 cloves garlic, minced
- 1 can (14 oz) crushed tomatoes
- 2 cups chicken broth
- Hot sauce to taste
- 1 cup frozen lima beans
- 1 cup frozen corn kernels
- 1 tablespoon Worcestershire sauce
- 1 teaspoon smoked paprika
- Salt and pepper to taste

INSTRUCTIONS:

1. Heat olive oil in a large pot over medium heat. Add onion and garlic, cooking until onion is translucent.
2. Add crushed tomatoes, chicken broth, lima beans, corn, Worcestershire sauce, and smoked paprika to the pot. Stir well to combine.
3. Bring to a boil, then reduce heat and simmer for about 45 minutes, or until vegetables are tender.
4. Stir in the shredded chicken and heat through. Season with salt, pepper, and hot sauce to taste.
5. Serve hot.

NUTRITIONAL INFORMATION (PER SERVING):

Calories: 300 | Carbs: 20g | Fiber: 5g | Net Carbs: 15g
Protein: 30g | Fats: 10g

Clam and Bacon Chowder

Prep Time: 15 Minutes | **Cook Time:** 30 Minutes | **Serves:** 4

INGREDIENTS:

- 4 slices bacon, chopped
- 1 onion, diced
- 2 cloves garlic, minced
- 2 cups cauliflower, chopped into small florets
- 1 cup heavy cream
- 2 cans (6.5 oz each) chopped clams, with juice
- 2 cups chicken or vegetable broth
- Salt and pepper to taste
- Fresh thyme for garnish

INSTRUCTIONS:

1. In a large pot, cook the bacon over medium heat until crisp. Remove bacon and set aside, leaving the grease in the pot.
2. Add onion and garlic to the bacon grease, and sauté until softened.
3. Add cauliflower and broth to the pot. Bring to a boil, then reduce heat and simmer until cauliflower is tender, about 15 minutes.
4. Stir in the clams with their juice and heavy cream. Heat through without boiling.
5. Season with salt and pepper to taste.
6. Serve the chowder garnished with crisp bacon pieces and fresh thyme.

NUTRITIONAL INFORMATION (PER SERVING):

Calories: 350 | Carbs: 8g | Fiber: 2g | Net Carbs: 6g
Protein: 15g | Fats: 28g

Beef Pho with Shirataki Noodles

Prep Time: 15 Minutes | **Cook Time:** 20 Minutes | **Serves:** 4

INGREDIENTS:

- 4 cups beef broth (homemade preferred for best flavor)
- 1 lb beef sirloin, thinly sliced
- 2 packs shirataki noodles, rinsed and drained
- 1 onion, thinly sliced
- 2 cloves garlic, minced
- 1 cinnamon stick
- 2 star anise
- 1 teaspoon fish sauce
- Bean sprouts, fresh basil, lime wedges, and sliced chili for garnish

INSTRUCTIONS:

1. In a large pot, bring the beef broth to a simmer with the cinnamon stick, star anise, onion, and garlic.
2. Add the fish sauce and simmer for 10 minutes to infuse the flavors.
3. Add the thinly sliced beef to the broth, and cook for about 2-3 minutes until just cooked through.
4. Divide the shirataki noodles among four bowls.
5. Pour the hot broth and beef over the noodles in each bowl.
6. Serve with bean sprouts, fresh basil, lime wedges, and sliced chili on the side for garnish.

NUTRITIONAL INFORMATION (PER SERVING):

Calories: 220 | Carbs: 5g | Fiber: 1g | Net Carbs: 4g
Protein: 25g | Fats: 10g

Taco Soup

Prep Time: 10 Minutes | **Cook Time:** 30 Minutes | **Serves:** 4

INGREDIENTS:

- 1 lb ground beef
- 1 onion, diced
- 2 cloves garlic, minced
- 1 can (14 oz) diced tomatoes, undrained
- 1 can (4 oz) green chilies, undrained
- 2 cups beef broth
- 2 tablespoons homemade or low-carb taco seasoning
- Salt and pepper to taste
- Sour cream, shredded cheese, and chopped cilantro for garnish

INSTRUCTIONS:

1. In a large pot, brown the ground beef over medium heat. Drain excess fat.
2. Add onion and garlic to the pot with the beef, and sauté until softened.
3. Stir in diced tomatoes, green chilies, beef broth, and taco seasoning. Bring to a boil.
4. Reduce heat and simmer for 20 minutes, allowing flavors to meld.
5. Season with salt and pepper to taste.
6. Serve hot, garnished with sour cream, shredded cheese, and chopped cilantro.

NUTRITIONAL INFORMATION (PER SERVING):

Calories: 300 | Carbs: 8g | Fiber: 2g | Net Carbs: 6g
Protein: 25g | Fats: 18g

Ham and Potato Chowder

Prep Time: 15 Minutes | **Cook Time:** 30 Minutes | **Serves:** 4

INGREDIENTS:

- 2 cups cauliflower florets, chopped into small pieces (as a low-carb potato substitute)
- 1 tablespoon olive oil
- 1 onion, diced
- 2 cloves garlic, minced
- 1 cup cooked ham, diced
- 3 cups chicken broth
- 1 cup heavy cream
- Salt and pepper to taste
- Fresh chives, chopped for garnish

INSTRUCTIONS:

1. In a large pot, heat olive oil over medium heat. Add onion and garlic, sautéing until softened.
2. Add the chopped cauliflower and diced ham to the pot. Cook for a few minutes until the cauliflower starts to soften.
3. Pour in the chicken broth and bring the mixture to a boil. Reduce heat and simmer for about 20 minutes, or until the cauliflower is tender.
4. Stir in the heavy cream and heat through. Do not boil.
5. Season with salt and pepper to taste.
6. Serve hot, garnished with fresh chives.

Calories: 300 | Carbs: 8g | Fiber: 2g | Net Carbs: 6g
Protein: 15g | Fats: 22g

Cioppino (Italian Fish Stew)

Prep Time: 20 Minutes | **Cook Time:** 40 Minutes
Serves: 4

INGREDIENTS:

- 2 tablespoons olive oil
- 1 onion, chopped
- 2 cloves garlic, minced
- 1 bell pepper, diced
- 1 can (14 oz) diced tomatoes
- 2 cups fish or vegetable broth
- Fresh parsley, chopped for garnish
- 1/2 cup dry white wine (optional, can be omitted for a lower carb option)
- 1 lb mixed seafood (shrimp, scallops, mussels, and firm white fish), cleaned and prepped
- Salt and pepper to taste

INSTRUCTIONS:

1. Heat olive oil in a large pot over medium heat. Add onion, garlic, and bell pepper, sautéing until softened.
2. Stir in diced tomatoes, broth, and white wine (if using). Bring to a simmer and cook for about 20 minutes.
3. Add the mixed seafood to the pot, ensuring that it is submerged in the liquid. Cover and cook for about 10 minutes, or until seafood is cooked through and mussels have opened.
4. Season with salt and pepper to taste.
5. Serve hot, garnished with fresh parsley.

NUTRITIONAL INFORMATION (PER SERVING):

Calories: 250 | Carbs: 10g | Fiber: 2g | Net Carbs: 8g
Protein: 25g | Fats: 10g

Thai Coconut Shrimp Soup

Prep Time: 15 Minutes | **Cook Time:** 20 Minutes
Serves: 4

INGREDIENTS:

- 1 tablespoon coconut oil
- 1 onion, diced
- 2 cloves garlic, minced
- 1 tablespoon fresh ginger, grated
- 1 tablespoon red curry paste
- 1 can (14 oz) coconut milk
- 2 cups chicken or vegetable broth
- 1 lb shrimp, peeled and deveined
- 1 cup mushrooms, sliced
- Juice of 1 lime
- Salt to taste
- Fresh cilantro for garnish

INSTRUCTIONS:

1. Heat coconut oil in a large pot over medium heat. Add onion, garlic, and ginger, cooking until softened.
2. Stir in red curry paste and cook for 1 minute until fragrant.
3. Add coconut milk and broth to the pot. Bring to a simmer.
4. Add shrimp and mushrooms to the soup. Simmer for about 5-7 minutes, or until shrimp are pink and cooked through.
5. Stir in lime juice and season with salt to taste.
6. Serve hot, garnished with fresh cilantro.

NUTRITIONAL INFORMATION (PER SERVING):

Calories: 300 | Carbs: 8g | Fiber: 1g | Net Carbs: 7g
Protein: 25g | Fats: 18g

Moroccan Lamb and Chickpea Stew

Prep Time: 20 Minutes | **Cook Time:** 90 Minutes
Serves: 4

INGREDIENTS:

- 1 lb lamb shoulder, cut into 1-inch cubes
- 2 tablespoons olive oil
- 1 onion, diced
- 2 cloves garlic, minced
- 1 teaspoon ground cumin
- 1 teaspoon ground cinnamon
- 2 cups beef broth

*   1/2 teaspoon ground ginger
*   1 can (14 oz) chickpeas, drained and rinsed (use low-carb beans for a lower carb option)
*   1 can (14 oz) diced tomatoes
*   Salt and pepper to taste
*   Fresh cilantro, chopped for garnish

1. Heat olive oil in a large pot over medium-high heat. Add lamb cubes and brown on all sides. Remove lamb and set aside.
2. In the same pot, add onion and garlic, cooking until softened.
3. Return lamb to the pot. Stir in cumin, cinnamon, and ginger.
4. Add diced tomatoes and beef broth. Bring to a boil, then reduce heat, cover, and simmer for 1 hour.
5. Stir in chickpeas and continue to simmer, uncovered, for an additional 30 minutes, or until the lamb is tender.
6. Season with salt and pepper to taste.
7. Serve hot, garnished with fresh cilantro.

NUTRITIONAL INFORMATION (PER SERVING):

Calories: 400 | Carbs: 10g | Fiber: 3g | Net Carbs: 7g
Protein: 35g | Fats: 28g

Tomato Basil Soup with Ricotta Dumplings

Prep Time: 20 Minutes | **Cook Time:** 30 Minutes |
Serves: 4

INGREDIENTS:

Ingredients for Soup:

*   2 tablespoons olive oil
*   1 onion, diced
*   2 cloves garlic, minced
*   1 can (28 oz) crushed tomatoes
*   2 cups vegetable broth

Ingredients for Ricotta Dumplings:

*   1 cup ricotta cheese
*   1/4 cup grated Parmesan cheese
*   1 egg
*   1/4 cup almond flour
*   Salt and pepper to taste

*   1/4 cup fresh basil, chopped
*   Salt and pepper to taste

INSTRUCTIONS:

1. Heat olive oil in a large pot over medium heat. Add onion and garlic, cooking until softened.
2. Stir in crushed tomatoes and vegetable broth. Bring to a boil, then reduce heat and simmer for 20 minutes.
3. While the soup simmers, mix together ricotta, Parmesan, egg, almond flour, salt, and pepper in a bowl to form the dumpling mixture.
4. Drop spoonfuls of the dumpling mixture into the simmering soup. Cook for an additional 10 minutes, or until dumplings are set.
5. Stir in fresh basil and season the soup with salt and pepper to taste.
6. Serve hot.

NUTRITIONAL INFORMATION (PER SERVING):

Calories: 300 | Carbs: 15g | Fiber: 4g | Net Carbs: 11g
Protein: 15g | Fats: 20g

Vegetable Beef Soup

Prep Time: 20 Minutes | **Cook Time:** 1 Hour |
Serves: 4

INGREDIENTS:

*   1 lb beef stew meat, cut into 1-inch cubes
*   2 tablespoons olive oil
*   1 onion, chopped
*   2 cloves garlic, minced
*   2 carrots, chopped
*   2 stalks celery, chopped
*   1 cup green beans, cut into 1-inch pieces
*   4 cups beef broth
*   1 can (14 oz) diced tomatoes
*   1 teaspoon dried thyme
*   Salt and pepper to taste
*   Fresh parsley, chopped for garnish

INSTRUCTIONS:

1. Heat olive oil in a large pot over medium-high heat. Add beef cubes and brown on all sides. Remove beef and set aside.
2. In the same pot, add onion, garlic, carrots, and celery, cooking until softened.

3. Return beef to the pot along with green beans, beef broth, diced tomatoes, and thyme.
4. Bring to a boil, then reduce heat, cover, and simmer for about 1 hour, or until the beef is tender and the vegetables are cooked.
5. Season with salt and pepper to taste.
6. Serve hot, garnished with fresh parsley.

NUTRITIONAL INFORMATION (PER SERVING):

Calories: 350 | Carbs: 12g | Fiber: 3g | Net Carbs: 9g
Protein: 35g | Fats: 18g

Spicy Pork and Cabbage Soup

Prep Time: 15 Minutes | **Cook Time:** 30 Minutes | **Serves:** 4

INGREDIENTS:

- ❖ 1 lb ground pork
- ❖ 2 tablespoons olive oil
- ❖ 2 cloves garlic, minced
- ❖ 1 teaspoon red pepper flakes (adjust to taste)
- ❖ 1 onion, diced
- ❖ 4 cups chicken broth
- ❖ 2 cups cabbage, shredded
- ❖ Salt and pepper to taste
- ❖ Fresh cilantro, chopped for garnish

INSTRUCTIONS:

1. Heat olive oil in a large pot over medium heat. Add the ground pork, breaking it apart with a spoon, and cook until browned.
2. Add onion, garlic, and red pepper flakes to the pot. Cook until the onion is softened.
3. Pour in the chicken broth and bring the mixture to a boil.
4. Add the shredded cabbage to the pot. Reduce heat and simmer for about 20 minutes, or until the cabbage is tender.
5. Season with salt and pepper to taste.
6. Serve the soup hot, garnished with fresh cilantro.

NUTRITIONAL INFORMATION (PER SERVING):

Calories: 300 | Carbs: 6g | Fiber: 2g | Net Carbs: 4g
Protein: 20g | Fats: 22g

Cauliflower Leek Soup

Prep Time: 10 Minutes | **Cook Time:** 25 Minutes | **Serves:** 4

INGREDIENTS:

- ❖ 1 large leek, white and light green parts only, sliced and washed
- ❖ 1 head cauliflower, cut into florets
- ❖ 2 tablespoons olive oil
- ❖ 4 cups vegetable broth
- ❖ 1 cup heavy cream
- ❖ Salt and pepper to taste
- ❖ Chives, chopped for garnish

INSTRUCTIONS:

1. Heat olive oil in a large pot over medium heat. Add the leeks and cook until softened, about 5 minutes.
2. Add the cauliflower florets and vegetable broth to the pot. Bring to a boil, then reduce heat and simmer until cauliflower is tender, about 15 minutes.
3. Use an immersion blender to puree the soup until smooth.
4. Stir in the heavy cream and heat through. Season with salt and pepper to taste.
5. Serve hot, garnished with chopped chives.

NUTRITIONAL INFORMATION (PER SERVING):

Calories: 280 | Carbs: 10g | Fiber: 3g | Net Carbs: 7g
Protein: 5g | Fats: 24g

Chapter 9

Vegetables and Sides

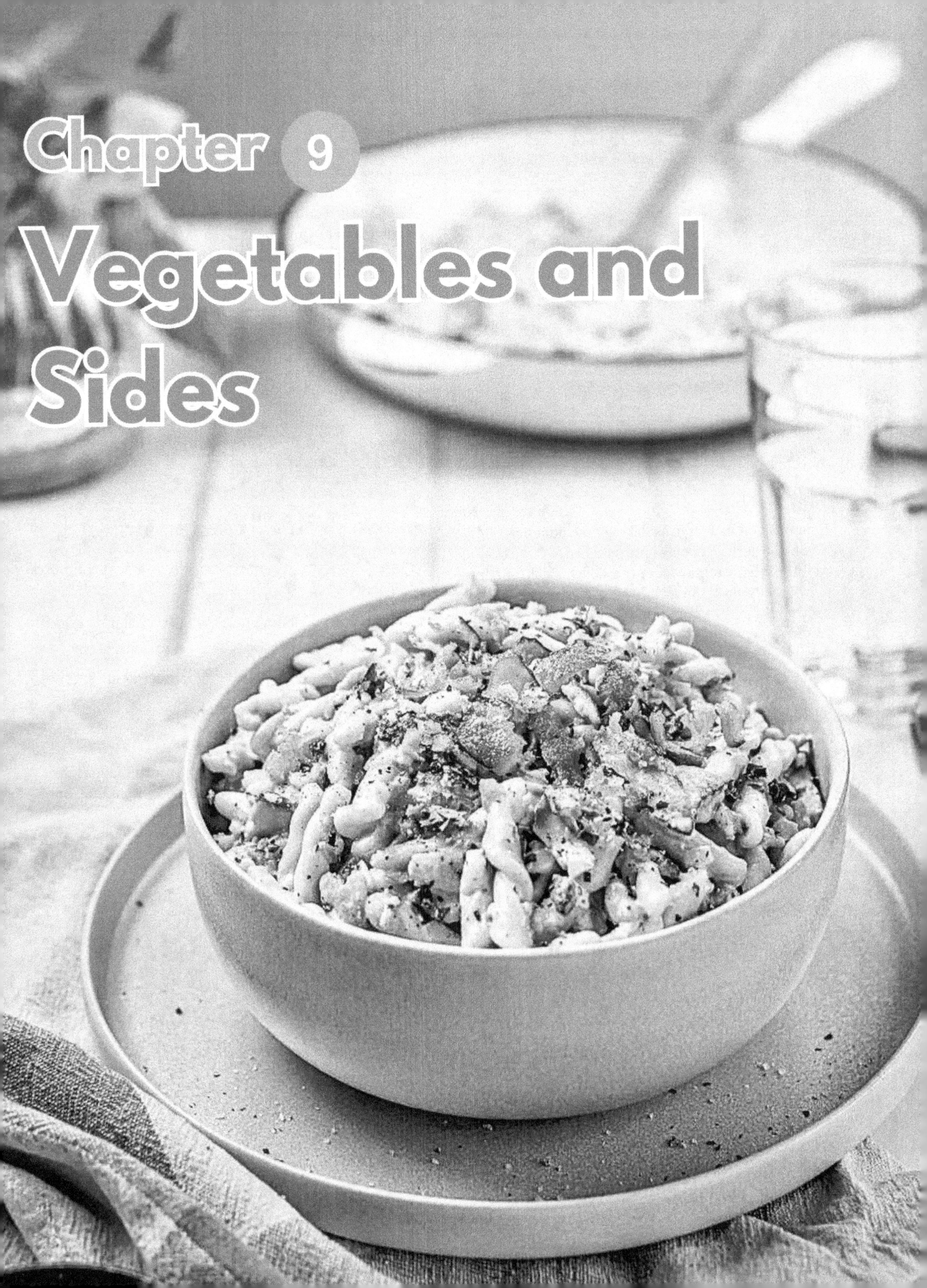

Cauliflower Rice Pilaf

Prep Time: 10 Minutes | **Cook Time:** 15 Minutes | **Serves:** 4

INGREDIENTS:

- 1 large head cauliflower, riced
- 2 tablespoons olive oil
- 1 onion, finely diced
- 2 cloves garlic, minced
- 1/4 cup almonds, slivered
- 1/4 cup dried cranberries (optional, omit for lower carbs)
- 1/4 cup fresh parsley, chopped
- Salt and pepper to taste

INSTRUCTIONS:

1. Heat olive oil in a large skillet over medium heat. Add onion and garlic, cooking until softened.
2. Add the riced cauliflower to the skillet. Cook, stirring occasionally, until the cauliflower is tender and slightly browned, about 10 minutes.
3. Stir in almonds and dried cranberries (if using). Cook for an additional 2-3 minutes.
4. Remove from heat and stir in fresh parsley. Season with salt and pepper to taste.
5. Serve hot as a side dish.

NUTRITIONAL INFORMATION (PER SERVING):

Calories: 180 | Carbs: 10g | Fiber: 4g | Net Carbs: 6g
Protein: 5g | Fats: 14g

Roasted Brussels Sprouts with Bacon

Prep Time: 10 Minutes | **Cook Time:** 25 Minutes | **Serves:** 4

INGREDIENTS:

- 1 lb Brussels sprouts, trimmed and halved
- 4 slices bacon, chopped
- 2 tablespoons olive oil
- Salt and pepper to taste

INSTRUCTIONS:

1. Preheat oven to 400°F (200°C).
2. In a large mixing bowl, toss the Brussels sprouts with olive oil, salt, and pepper.
3. Spread the Brussels sprouts on a baking sheet in a single layer. Sprinkle the chopped bacon over the top.
4. Roast in the preheated oven for about 25 minutes, or until the Brussels sprouts are tender and caramelized, and the bacon is crispy.
5. Serve hot as a side dish.

NUTRITIONAL INFORMATION (PER SERVING):

Calories: 180 | Carbs: 10g | Fiber: 4g | Net Carbs: 6g
Protein: 8g | Fats: 12g

Garlic Parmesan Green Beans

Prep Time: 5 Minutes | **Cook Time:** 15 Minutes | **Serves:** 4

INGREDIENTS:

- 1 lb green beans, trimmed
- 2 tablespoons olive oil
- 2 cloves garlic, minced
- 1/4 cup grated Parmesan cheese
- Salt and pepper to taste

INSTRUCTIONS:

1. Heat olive oil in a large skillet over medium heat. Add the minced garlic and sauté for about 1 minute, until fragrant.
2. Add the green beans to the skillet. Cook, stirring occasionally, for about 10-12 minutes, or until the green beans are tender but still crisp.
3. Remove from heat and sprinkle with grated Parmesan cheese. Season with salt and pepper to taste.
4. Toss everything together until the green beans are evenly coated with the cheese.
5. Serve hot as a side dish.

NUTRITIONAL INFORMATION (PER SERVING):

Calories: 120 | Carbs: 8g | Fiber: 3g | Net Carbs: 5g
Protein: 5g | Fats: 8g

Zucchini Fritters

Prep Time: 20 Minutes | **Cook Time:** 10 Minutes |
Serves: 4

INGREDIENTS:

- 2 medium zucchinis, grated
- 1 teaspoon salt (for draining zucchini)
- 2 eggs, beaten
- 1/2 cup almond flour
- 1/4 cup grated Parmesan cheese
- 2 tablespoons fresh chives, chopped
- 1 clove garlic, minced
- Salt and pepper to taste
- 2 tablespoons olive oil for frying

INSTRUCTIONS:

1. Place the grated zucchini in a colander, sprinkle with 1 teaspoon salt, and let it sit for 10 minutes to draw out moisture. Squeeze out the excess water.
2. In a bowl, combine the drained zucchini, beaten eggs, almond flour, Parmesan cheese, chives, minced garlic, salt, and pepper. Mix well to form a batter.
3. Heat olive oil in a large skillet over medium heat. Scoop spoonfuls of the zucchini mixture into the skillet, flattening them slightly to form fritters.
4. Fry for about 4-5 minutes on each side, or until golden brown and crispy.
5. Serve hot, either as a side dish or a light main course.

NUTRITIONAL INFORMATION (PER SERVING):

Calories: 200 | Carbs: 8g | Fiber: 3g | Net Carbs: 5g
Protein: 10g | Fats: 14g

Creamed Spinach

Prep Time: 10 Minutes | **Cook Time:** 15 Minutes |
Serves: 4

INGREDIENTS:

- 2 tablespoons unsalted butter
- 1 small onion, finely chopped
- 2 cloves garlic, minced
- 10 ounces fresh spinach, washed and trimmed
- 1/2 cup heavy cream
- 1/4 cup grated Parmesan cheese
- Salt and nutmeg to taste
- Black pepper to taste

INSTRUCTIONS:

1. In a large skillet, melt butter over medium heat. Add onion and garlic, sautéing until translucent and fragrant.
2. Gradually add spinach to the skillet, stirring until wilted. You may need to add the spinach in batches.
3. Stir in heavy cream and simmer for a few minutes until the mixture thickens slightly.
4. Add Parmesan cheese, salt, nutmeg, and black pepper. Stir until the cheese is melted and the mixture is well combined.
5. Serve hot as a side dish.

NUTRITIONAL INFORMATION (PER SERVING):

Calories: 180 | Carbs: 5g | Fiber: 2g | Net Carbs: 3g
Protein: 5g | Fats: 16g

Radish Chips

Prep Time: 10 Minutes | **Cook Time:** 20 Minutes |
Serves: 4

INGREDIENTS:

- 20 radishes, thinly sliced
- Salt and pepper to taste
- 1 tablespoon olive oil
- Optional seasonings: garlic powder, paprika, or dried herbs

INSTRUCTIONS:

1. Preheat your oven to 375°F (190°C). Line a baking sheet with parchment paper.
2. In a bowl, toss the thinly sliced radishes with olive oil, salt, pepper, and any additional seasonings you like.
3. Spread the radish slices in a single layer on the prepared baking sheet.
4. Bake in the preheated oven for 10 minutes, then flip the slices and bake for another 10 minutes or until crispy.
5. Serve hot or at room temperature as a snack or side dish.

NUTRITIONAL INFORMATION (PER SERVING):

Calories: 45 | Carbs: 2g | Fiber: 1g | Net Carbs: 1g
Protein: 1g | Fats: 4g

Eggplant Parmesan Stacks

Prep Time: 20 Minutes | **Cook Time:** 30 Minutes | **Serves:** 4

INGREDIENTS:

- 2 medium eggplants, sliced into 1/2-inch rounds
- 2 tablespoons olive oil
- 1 cup low-carb marinara sauce
- Salt and pepper to taste
- 1 cup shredded mozzarella cheese
- 1/4 cup grated Parmesan cheese
- Fresh basil leaves for garnish

INSTRUCTIONS:

1. Preheat your oven to 400°F (200°C). Line a baking sheet with parchment paper.
2. Arrange eggplant slices on the baking sheet. Brush both sides with olive oil and season with salt and pepper.
3. Bake for 15-20 minutes, flipping halfway through, until eggplant is tender and slightly browned.
4. On a separate baking sheet or in a baking dish, create eggplant stacks by layering an eggplant slice, a spoonful of marinara sauce, a sprinkle of mozzarella, and another eggplant slice. Repeat layers and top with Parmesan cheese.
5. Bake for an additional 10 minutes, or until cheese is melted and bubbly.
6. Serve hot, garnished with fresh basil leaves.

NUTRITIONAL INFORMATION (PER SERVING):

Calories: 250 | Carbs: 12g | Fiber: 5g | Net Carbs: 7g
Protein: 12g | Fats: 18g

Green Beans with Red Peppers

Prep Time: 10 Minutes | **Cook Time:** 15 Minutes | **Serves:** 4

INGREDIENTS:

- 1 lb fresh green beans, trimmed
- 2 tablespoons olive oil
- 1 red bell pepper, sliced into thin strips
- 2 cloves garlic, minced
- Salt and pepper to taste
- Lemon zest for garnish (optional)

INSTRUCTIONS:

1. Bring a large pot of salted water to a boil. Add green beans and cook for about 3-4 minutes until crisp-tender. Drain and immediately plunge into ice water to stop the cooking process. Drain again.
2. Heat olive oil in a large skillet over medium heat. Add red bell pepper strips and sauté until they start to soften, about 5 minutes.
3. Add minced garlic to the skillet and cook for another minute until fragrant.
4. Add the blanched green beans to the skillet. Toss to combine and heat through. Season with salt and pepper.
5. Serve hot, garnished with lemon zest if desired.

NUTRITIONAL INFORMATION (PER SERVING):

Calories: 110 | Carbs: 8g | Fiber: 3g | Net Carbs: 5g
Protein: 2g | Fats: 8g

Balsamic Roasted Vegetables

Prep Time: 15 Minutes | **Cook Time:** 25 Minutes | **Serves:** 4

INGREDIENTS:

- 2 cups broccoli florets
- 2 cups cauliflower florets
- 1 red onion, cut into wedges
- 2 carrots, sliced
- 2 tablespoons olive oil
- 2 tablespoons balsamic vinegar
- Salt and pepper to taste
- Fresh thyme leaves for garnish (optional)

INSTRUCTIONS:

1. Preheat your oven to 425°F (220°C). Line a large baking sheet with parchment paper.
2. In a large bowl, combine broccoli, cauliflower, red onion, and carrots. Drizzle with olive oil and balsamic vinegar. Toss to coat evenly.
3. Spread the vegetables in a single layer on the prepared baking sheet. Season with salt and pepper.

4. Roast in the preheated oven for 25 minutes, or until vegetables are tender and caramelized, stirring halfway through.
5. Serve hot, garnished with fresh thyme leaves if desired.

Calories: 130 | Carbs: 12g | Fiber:4g | Net Carbs: 8g
Protein: 3g | Fats: 8g

Spaghetti Squash Alfredo

Prep Time: 10 Minutes | **Cook Time:** 40 Minutes | **Serves:** 4

INGREDIENTS:

- 1 large spaghetti squash
- 2 tablespoons unsalted butter
- 1/2 cup grated Parmesan cheese
- 1 cup heavy cream
- 1 clove garlic, minced
- Salt and pepper to taste
- Fresh parsley, chopped for garnish

INSTRUCTIONS:

1. Preheat your oven to 400°F (200°C). Halve the spaghetti squash lengthwise and scoop out the seeds.
2. Place the squash halves cut-side down on a baking sheet. Roast for 30-40 minutes, or until tender.
3. Use a fork to scrape the squash strands into a bowl, creating "spaghetti."
4. In a saucepan, melt butter over medium heat. Add garlic and sauté until fragrant.
5. Stir in heavy cream and bring to a simmer. Reduce heat and add Parmesan cheese, stirring until melted and the sauce is smooth.
6. Combine the spaghetti squash strands with the Alfredo sauce. Toss to coat evenly. Season with salt and pepper.
7. Serve hot, garnished with fresh parsley.

NUTRITIONAL INFORMATION (PER SERVING):

Calories: 350 | Carbs: 10g | Fiber:2g | Net Carbs: 8g
Protein: 7g | Fats: 32g

Kale and Avocado Salad

Prep Time: 15 Minutes | **Cook Time:** 0 Minutes | **Serves:** 4

INGREDIENTS:

- 4 cups kale, stems removed and leaves chopped
- 1/4 cup red onion, thinly sliced
- 1/2 cup cherry tomatoes, halved
- 1/4 cup almonds, slivered
- 1 ripe avocado, diced
- 2 tablespoons olive oil
- 1 tablespoon lemon juice
- Salt and pepper to taste
- Parmesan cheese shavings for garnish (optional)

INSTRUCTIONS:

1. In a large bowl, combine the chopped kale, diced avocado, sliced red onion, cherry tomatoes, and slivered almonds.
2. In a small bowl, whisk together the olive oil and lemon juice. Season with salt and pepper.
3. Pour the dressing over the salad and toss well to ensure all the ingredients are evenly coated.
4. Let the salad sit for about 5 minutes to allow the kale to soften slightly.
5. Serve garnished with Parmesan cheese shavings if desired.

NUTRITIONAL INFORMATION (PER SERVING):

Calories: 250 | Carbs: 12g | Fiber: 6g | Net Carbs: 6g
Protein: 6g | Fats: 20g

Simple Bibimbap

Prep Time: 20 Minutes | **Cook Time:** 20 Minutes | **Serves:** 4

INGREDIENTS:

- 2 cups cauliflower rice (as a low-carb substitute for traditional rice)
- 1 tablespoon sesame oil
- 1/2 lb ground beef or turkey
- 1 cup spinach, sautéed
- 1 cup mushrooms, sautéed

- ❖ 2 tablespoons low-sodium soy sauce or tamari
- ❖ 1 tablespoon gochujang (Korean chili paste, adjust to taste)
- ❖ 1 carrot, julienned
- ❖ 4 eggs
- ❖ Sesame seeds for garnish
- ❖ Green onions, chopped for garnish

INSTRUCTIONS:

1. Prepare cauliflower rice by pulsing cauliflower florets in a food processor until it resembles rice grains. Sauté in a pan with a little sesame oil until tender.
2. In another pan, cook the ground beef or turkey with a bit of sesame oil until fully cooked. Set aside.
3. Sauté spinach and mushrooms in separate pans until tender. Set aside.
4. Julienne the carrot and set aside.
5. Fry the eggs to your preference (sunny side up is traditional).
6. Assemble the bibimbap by placing a portion of cauliflower rice in each bowl. Arrange the ground meat, spinach, mushrooms, and carrot over the rice.
7. Top each bowl with a fried egg.
8. Mix soy sauce or tamari with gochujang and drizzle over each bowl.
9. Garnish with sesame seeds and chopped green onions.
10. Stir everything together before eating.

NUTRITIONAL INFORMATION (PER SERVING):

Calories: 350 | Carbs: 12g | Fiber: 3g | Net Carbs: 9g
Protein: 25g | Fats: 22g

Ratatouille

Prep Time: 20 Minutes | **Cook Time:** 40 Minutes |
Serves: 4

INGREDIENTS:

- ❖ 1 eggplant, sliced
- ❖ 2 zucchinis, sliced
- ❖ 1 yellow squash, sliced
- ❖ 1 red bell pepper, sliced
- ❖ 2 tomatoes, sliced
- ❖ 1/4 cup olive oil
- ❖ 2 cloves garlic, minced
- ❖ 1 teaspoon thyme
- ❖ Salt and pepper to taste
- ❖ Fresh basil for garnish

INSTRUCTIONS:

1. Preheat your oven to 375°F (190°C).
2. In a baking dish, spread a thin layer of olive oil and sprinkle minced garlic and thyme.
3. Arrange the sliced vegetables in the dish, alternating and overlapping them (eggplant, zucchini, yellow squash, bell pepper, tomato).
4. Drizzle the remaining olive oil over the vegetables and season with salt and pepper.
5. Cover the dish with foil and bake for 30 minutes. Remove the foil and bake for an additional 10 minutes or until the vegetables are tender.
6. Garnish with fresh basil before serving.

NUTRITIONAL INFORMATION (PER SERVING):

Calories: 180 | Carbs: 15g | Fiber: 6g | Net Carbs: 9g
Protein: 3g | Fats: 14g

Summer Squash Casserole

Prep Time: 15 Minutes | **Cook Time:** 30 Minutes |
Serves: 4

INGREDIENTS:

- ❖ 2 medium zucchinis, sliced
- ❖ 2 medium yellow squash, sliced
- ❖ 1/2 cup almond flour
- ❖ 1/2 cup grated Parmesan cheese
- ❖ 2 eggs, beaten
- ❖ 1/4 cup heavy cream
- ❖ 1/2 teaspoon garlic powder
- ❖ Salt and pepper to taste
- ❖ 1/2 cup shredded mozzarella cheese
- ❖ Fresh parsley, chopped for garnish

INSTRUCTIONS:

1. Preheat your oven to 375°F (190°C). Grease a baking dish.
2. In a bowl, mix together almond flour, Parmesan cheese, garlic powder, salt, and pepper.
3. In another bowl, whisk together the beaten eggs and heavy cream.
4. Layer half of the sliced zucchini and yellow squash in the bottom of the baking dish. Sprinkle with half of the almond flour mixture.
5. Pour half of the egg and cream mixture over the top.
6. Repeat the layers with the remaining zucchini, yellow

squash, almond flour mixture, and egg mixture.

7. Top with shredded mozzarella cheese.
8. Bake in the preheated oven for 30 minutes, or until the top is golden and bubbly.
9. Garnish with fresh parsley before serving.

NUTRITIONAL INFORMATION (PER SERVING):

Calories: 280 | Carbs: 10g | Fiber: 4g | Net Carbs: 6g
Protein: 18g | Fats: 20g

Sautéed Mushrooms with Thyme

Prep Time: 5 Minutes | **Cook Time:** 10 Minutes |
Serves: 4

INGREDIENTS:

- 1 lb mushrooms, cleaned and sliced
- 2 tablespoons butter
- 2 cloves garlic, minced
- 1 teaspoon fresh thyme leaves
- Salt and pepper to taste

INSTRUCTIONS:

1. Melt butter in a large skillet over medium heat.
2. Add the sliced mushrooms and sauté until they are golden and their liquid has evaporated, about 5-7 minutes.
3. Add minced garlic and thyme leaves, cooking for another 2-3 minutes until fragrant.
4. Season with salt and pepper to taste.
5. Serve hot as a side dish.

NUTRITIONAL INFORMATION (PER SERVING):

Calories: 100 | Carbs: 4g | Fiber: 1g | Net Carbs: 3g
Protein: 3g | Fats: 8g

Herb-Roasted Root Vegetables

Prep Time: 15 Minutes | **Cook Time:** 35 Minutes |
Serves: 4

INGREDIENTS:

- 2 carrots, peeled and chopped
- 2 parsnips, peeled and chopped
- 1 sweet potato, peeled and chopped
- 1 beet, peeled and chopped
- 2 tablespoons olive oil
- 1 teaspoon rosemary, chopped
- 1 teaspoon thyme, chopped
- Salt and pepper to taste

INSTRUCTIONS:

1. Start by preheating your oven to 400°F (200°C).
2. In a large bowl, combine the chopped carrots, parsnips, sweet potato, and beet.
3. Drizzle with olive oil and sprinkle with rosemary, thyme, salt, and pepper. Toss to coat evenly.
4. Spread the vegetables in a single layer on a baking sheet.
5. Roast in the preheated oven for 35 minutes, or until the vegetables are tender and caramelized, stirring occasionally.
6. Serve hot as a side dish.

NUTRITIONAL INFORMATION (PER SERVING):

Calories: 180 | Carbs: 24g | Fiber: 6g | Net Carbs: 18g
Protein: 2g | Fats: 9g

Cheesy Broccoli Casserole

Prep Time: 10 Minutes | **Cook Time:** 20 Minutes |
Serves: 4

INGREDIENTS:

- 4 cups broccoli florets
- 1 cup heavy cream
- 1 cup shredded cheddar cheese
- 1/2 cup cream cheese
- 1 teaspoon garlic powder
- 1/4 cup chicken broth
- Salt and pepper to taste
- 1/4 cup grated Parmesan cheese for topping

INSTRUCTIONS:

1. Preheat your oven to 375°F (190°C).
2. Steam broccoli florets until just tender, about 3-4 minutes, then drain any excess water.
3. In a saucepan over medium heat, combine heavy cream, cheddar cheese, cream cheese, chicken broth, and garlic powder. Stir until the cheeses are melted and the

mixture is smooth.

4. Season with salt and pepper to taste.
5. Mix the steamed broccoli into the cheese sauce, then transfer the mixture to a baking dish.
6. Sprinkle grated Parmesan cheese on top.
7. Bake in the preheated oven for 15-20 minutes or until the top is golden and bubbly.
8. Serve hot as a side dish.

Calories: 350 | Carbs: 8g | Fiber: 2g | Net Carbs: 6g
Protein:12g | Fats: 30g

Stuffed Artichokes

Prep Time: 20 Minutes | **Cook Time:** 45 Minutes |
Serves: 4

INGREDIENTS:

- 4 large artichokes
- 1 cup almond flour
- 1/2 cup grated Parmesan cheese
- 2 cloves garlic, minced
- 2 tablespoons fresh parsley, chopped
- 1 lemon, juiced
- 2 tablespoons olive oil
- Salt and pepper to taste

INSTRUCTIONS:

1. Preheat your oven to 375°F (190°C).
2. Prepare the artichokes by trimming the stems and removing the tough outer leaves. Cut off the top third of each artichoke.
3. In a bowl, combine almond flour, Parmesan cheese, garlic, parsley, lemon juice, salt, and pepper.
4. Gently spread the leaves of each artichoke and stuff the almond flour mixture between them.
5. Place the artichokes in a baking dish and drizzle with olive oil. Add a little water to the bottom of the dish to prevent burning.
6. Cover with foil and bake for about 45 minutes, or until the artichokes are tender and the stuffing is golden.
7. Serve hot, allowing each person to pull off leaves and enjoy the stuffed artichoke.

NUTRITIONAL INFORMATION (PER SERVING):

Calories: 280 | Carbs: 18g | Fiber: 9g | Net Carbs: 9g
Protein:12g | Fats: 20g

Cucumber and Dill Salad

Prep Time: 10 Minutes | **Cook Time:** 0 Minutes |
Serves: 4

INGREDIENTS:

- 2 large cucumbers, thinly sliced
- 1/4 cup fresh dill, chopped
- 1/4 cup apple cider vinegar
- 2 tablespoons olive oil
- 1 tablespoon erythritol or other low-carb sweetener (optional)
- Salt and pepper to taste

INSTRUCTIONS:

1. In a large bowl, combine the thinly sliced cucumbers and chopped dill.
2. In a small bowl, whisk together apple cider vinegar, olive oil, erythritol (if using), salt, and pepper.
3. Pour the dressing over the cucumbers and dill, and toss to coat evenly.
4. Refrigerate for at least 30 minutes to allow the flavors to meld.
5. Serve chilled as a refreshing side dish.

NUTRITIONAL INFORMATION (PER SERVING):

Calories: 80 | Carbs: 4g | Fiber: 1g | Net Carbs: 3g
Protein: 1g | Fats: 7g

Grilled Asparagus with Lemon

Prep Time: 5 Minutes | **Cook Time:** 10 Minutes |
Serves: 4

INGREDIENTS:

- 1 lb fresh asparagus, trimmed
- 2 tablespoons olive oil
- Salt and pepper to taste
- 1 lemon, halved

INSTRUCTIONS:

1. Preheat your grill to medium-high heat.
2. Toss the asparagus spears with olive oil, salt, and pepper until evenly coated.
3. Place the asparagus on the grill in a single layer. Grill for about 10 minutes, turning occasionally, until the spears are tender and have grill marks.

4. Squeeze fresh lemon juice over the grilled asparagus just before serving.
5. Serve hot as a side dish.

Calories: 80 | Carbs: 5g | Fiber: 2g | Net Carbs: 3g | Protein: 3g | Fats: 6g

Roasted Radishes with Garlic and Rosemary

Prep Time: 10 Minutes | **Cook Time:** 25 Minutes | **Serves:** 4

INGREDIENTS:

- 1 lb radishes, trimmed and halved
- 2 tablespoons olive oil
- 2 cloves garlic, minced
- 1 tablespoon fresh rosemary, chopped
- Salt and pepper to taste

INSTRUCTIONS:

1. Preheat your oven to 400°F (200°C).
2. In a mixing bowl, toss the halved radishes with olive oil, minced garlic, chopped rosemary, salt, and pepper until well coated.
3. Spread the radishes out in a single layer on a baking sheet.
4. Roast in the preheated oven for 25 minutes, or until the radishes are tender and golden brown.
5. Serve hot as a flavorful side dish.

NUTRITIONAL INFORMATION (PER SERVING):

Calories: 70 | Carbs: 3g | Fiber: 1g | Net Carbs: 2g | Protein: 1g | Fats: 6g

Butternut Squash Fries

Prep Time: 15 Minutes | **Cook Time:** 30 Minutes | **Serves:** 4

INGREDIENTS:

- 1 medium butternut squash, peeled, seeded, and cut into fry-shaped strips
- 2 tablespoons olive oil
- Salt and pepper to taste
- **Optional spices:** paprika, garlic powder, or rosemary

INSTRUCTIONS:

1. Preheat your oven to 425°F (220°C). Line a baking sheet with parchment paper.
2. In a large bowl, toss the butternut squash strips with olive oil, salt, pepper, and any optional spices you're using until well coated.
3. Arrange the squash fries in a single layer on the prepared baking sheet, ensuring they're not touching for even cooking.
4. Bake in the preheated oven for about 30 minutes, turning halfway through, until the fries are golden and crispy.
5. Serve hot, possibly with a low-carb dipping sauce.

NUTRITIONAL INFORMATION (PER SERVING):

Calories: 120 | Carbs: 15g | Fiber: 2g | Net Carbs: 13g | Protein: 2g | Fats: 7g

Fennel and Chickpeas

Prep Time: 10 Minutes | **Cook Time:** 20 Minutes | **Serves:** 4

INGREDIENTS:

- 2 fennel bulbs, thinly sliced
- 1 can (14 oz) chickpeas, drained and rinsed
- 2 tablespoons olive oil
- 1 clove garlic, minced
- Salt and pepper to taste
- 1/4 cup grated Parmesan cheese
- Lemon wedges for serving

INSTRUCTIONS:

1. Heat olive oil in a large skillet over medium heat.
2. Add the sliced fennel and minced garlic to the skillet. Sauté until the fennel is tender and slightly caramelized, about 15 minutes.

3. Stir in the chickpeas and cook until heated through, about 5 minutes.
4. Season with salt and pepper to taste.
5. Sprinkle grated Parmesan cheese over the top just before serving.
6. Serve hot with lemon wedges on the side.

NUTRITIONAL INFORMATION (PER SERVING):

Calories: 220 | Carbs: 20g | Fiber: 6g | Net Carbs: 14g Protein: 8g | Fats: 12g

Creamy Cucumber Salad with Sour Cream and Dill

Prep Time: 15 Minutes | **Cook Time:** 0 Minutes | **Serves:** 4

INGREDIENTS:

- 2 large cucumbers, thinly sliced
- 1/2 cup sour cream
- 2 tablespoons fresh dill, chopped
- 1 tablespoon lemon juice
- 1 clove garlic, minced
- Salt and pepper to taste

INSTRUCTIONS:

1. In a large bowl, combine the sour cream, chopped dill, lemon juice, minced garlic, salt, and pepper. Mix until smooth.
2. Add the thinly sliced cucumbers to the bowl with the sour cream mixture. Toss gently to coat the cucumbers evenly.
3. Cover and refrigerate for at least 1 hour to allow the flavors to meld.
4. Serve chilled as a refreshing side dish.

NUTRITIONAL INFORMATION (PER SERVING):

Calories: 90 | Carbs: 6g | Fiber: 1g | Net Carbs: 5g Protein: 2g | Fats: 7g

Garlic Butter Sautéed Spinach

Prep Time: 5 Minutes | **Cook Time:** 5 Minutes | **Serves:** 4

INGREDIENTS:

- 1 lb fresh spinach leaves
- 2 tablespoons unsalted butter
- 2 cloves garlic, minced
- Salt and pepper to taste
- A squeeze of lemon juice (optional)

INSTRUCTIONS:

1. Heat butter in a large skillet over medium heat.
2. Add minced garlic to the skillet and sauté for about 30 seconds until fragrant.
3. Add the spinach leaves to the skillet. Cook, stirring frequently, until the spinach is wilted and tender, about 3-4 minutes.
4. Season with salt and pepper to taste. Add a squeeze of lemon juice if desired for extra flavor.
5. Serve hot as a nutritious and flavorful side dish.

NUTRITIONAL INFORMATION (PER SERVING):

Calories: 80 | Carbs: 4g | Fiber: 2g | Net Carbs: 2g Protein: 3g | Fats: 6g

Caprese Salad with Balsamic Reduction

Prep Time: 10 Minutes | **Cook Time:** 15 Minutes | **Serves:** 4

INGREDIENTS:

- 4 large ripe tomatoes, sliced
- 8 oz fresh mozzarella cheese, sliced
- 1/4 cup fresh basil leaves
- 1/2 cup balsamic vinegar
- 2 tablespoons olive oil
- Salt and pepper to taste

INSTRUCTIONS:

1. To make the balsamic reduction, pour balsamic vinegar into a small saucepan. Bring to a boil, then reduce heat to low and simmer until the vinegar thickens and reduces to about 1/4 cup, approximately 15 minutes. Allow it to cool.
2. Arrange the tomato and mozzarella slices alternately on a platter, overlapping them for presentation. Scatter fresh basil leaves over the top.
3. Drizzle olive oil and the balsamic reduction over the

arranged tomatoes and mozzarella.

4. Season with salt and pepper to taste.
5. Serve immediately as a fresh and flavorful appetizer or side dish.

Calories: 250 | Carbs: 8g | Fiber: 1g | Net Carbs: 7g
Protein: 15g | Fats: 18g

Grilled Portobello Mushrooms

Prep Time: 10 Minutes | **Cook Time:** 10 Minutes |
Serves: 4

INGREDIENTS:

- 4 large Portobello mushroom caps
- 2 tablespoons olive oil
- 2 cloves garlic, minced
- 1 tablespoon balsamic vinegar
- Salt and pepper to taste
- Fresh parsley, chopped for garnish

INSTRUCTIONS:

1. Preheat your grill to medium-high heat.
2. In a small bowl, whisk together olive oil, minced garlic, and balsamic vinegar.
3. Brush both sides of the Portobello mushrooms with the olive oil mixture and season with salt and pepper.
4. Grill the mushrooms for about 5 minutes on each side, or until they are tender and grill marks appear.
5. Garnish with fresh parsley before serving.
6. These grilled mushrooms can be served as a side dish or used as a meaty, vegetarian main course.

NUTRITIONAL INFORMATION (PER SERVING):

Calories: 100 | Carbs: 4g | Fiber: 1g | Net Carbs: 3g
Protein: 2g | Fats: 9g

Teriyaki Green Beans

Prep Time: 5 Minutes | **Cook Time:** 10 Minutes |
Serves: 4

INGREDIENTS:

- 1 lb green beans, trimmed
- 2 tablespoons low-sugar teriyaki sauce
- 1 tablespoon olive oil
- 1 teaspoon sesame seeds
- Salt to taste

INSTRUCTIONS:

1. Heat olive oil in a large skillet over medium heat.
2. Add the green beans and sauté for about 5 minutes, or until they start to become tender.
3. Pour the teriyaki sauce over the green beans and continue to cook for another 5 minutes, stirring occasionally, until the sauce thickens and coats the beans.
4. Season with salt to taste.
5. Sprinkle sesame seeds over the top before serving.
6. Serve hot as a flavorful side dish.

NUTRITIONAL INFORMATION (PER SERVING):

Calories: 80 | Carbs: 8g | Fiber: 3g | Net Carbs: 5g
Protein: 2g | Fats: 4g

Cauliflower Tabouleh

Prep Time: 15 Minutes | **Cook Time:** 0 Minutes |
Serves: 4

INGREDIENTS:

- 1 large head of cauliflower, riced
- 1 cup fresh parsley, finely chopped
- 1/2 cup fresh mint, finely chopped
- 2 tomatoes, diced
- 1 cucumber, diced
- 1/4 cup olive oil
- Juice of 1 lemon
- Salt and pepper to taste

INSTRUCTIONS:

1. Rice the cauliflower by pulsing cauliflower florets in a food processor until it resembles small grains. Transfer to a large mixing bowl.
2. Add the chopped parsley, mint, diced tomatoes, and cucumber to the bowl with the cauliflower rice.
3. In a small bowl, whisk together the olive oil and lemon juice. Pour this dressing over the cauliflower mixture.
4. Toss all the ingredients together until well combined. Season with salt and pepper to taste.

5. Refrigerate for at least 30 minutes before serving to allow the flavors to meld.
6. Serve chilled as a refreshing and healthy alternative to traditional tabouleh.

Calories: 180 | Carbs: 12g | Fiber: 4g | Net Carbs: 8g Protein: 4g | Fats: 14g

Lemon Parmesan Roasted Broccoli

Prep Time: 10 Minutes | **Cook Time:** 20 Minutes | **Serves:** 4

INGREDIENTS:

- ❖ 4 cups broccoli florets
- ❖ 2 tablespoons olive oil
- ❖ Juice and zest of 1 lemon
- ❖ 1/4 cup grated Parmesan cheese
- ❖ Salt and pepper to taste

INSTRUCTIONS:

1. Preheat your oven to 400°F (200°C).
2. In a large mixing bowl, toss the broccoli florets with olive oil, lemon juice, and half of the lemon zest. Season with salt and pepper.
3. Spread the broccoli in a single layer on a baking sheet.
4. Roast in the preheated oven for about 20 minutes, or until the broccoli is tender and the edges are crispy.
5. Remove from the oven and sprinkle with grated Parmesan cheese and the remaining lemon zest.
6. Serve hot as a flavorful and nutritious side dish.

NUTRITIONAL INFORMATION (PER SERVING):

Calories: 120 | Carbs: 6g | Fiber: 2g | Net Carbs: 4g Protein: 5g | Fats: 9g

Green Bean Almondine

Prep Time: 10 Minutes | **Cook Time:** 10 Minutes | **Serves:** 4

INGREDIENTS:

- ❖ 1 lb green beans, trimmed
- ❖ 2 tablespoons unsalted butter
- ❖ 1/2 cup sliced almonds
- ❖ 2 cloves garlic, minced
- ❖ Salt and pepper to taste
- ❖ Lemon wedges for serving

INSTRUCTIONS:

1. Bring a large pot of salted water to a boil. Add the green beans and cook for about 3-4 minutes until bright green and tender-crisp. Drain and plunge into ice water to stop the cooking process. Drain again.
2. In a large skillet, melt the butter over medium heat. Add the sliced almonds and garlic, sautéing until the almonds are golden and fragrant.
3. Add the blanched green beans to the skillet. Toss to coat with the butter and almond mixture. Season with salt and pepper.
4. Cook for an additional 2-3 minutes, until the green beans are heated through.
5. Serve hot, garnished with lemon wedges on the side.

NUTRITIONAL INFORMATION (PER SERVING):

Calories: 180 | Carbs: 8g | Fiber: 4g | Net Carbs: 4g Protein: 5g | Fats: 15g

<u>DOWNLOAD YOUR FREE GIFT NOW!</u>

As a thank you gesture, we're providing you free access to four essential meal planning tools: a weekly meal planner, a beautifully designed recipe card, a grocery shopping list, and a food journal. These tools are not just practical aids; they're your cooking companion, providing structure, inspiration, and organization. To gain access, simply scan the QR code provided below.

Enjoying this book? Discover more of our books from our Amazon author page. Scan the QR code below to purchase a variety of similar books, expanding your culinary repertoire with every page.

Chapter 10
Vegetarian Mains

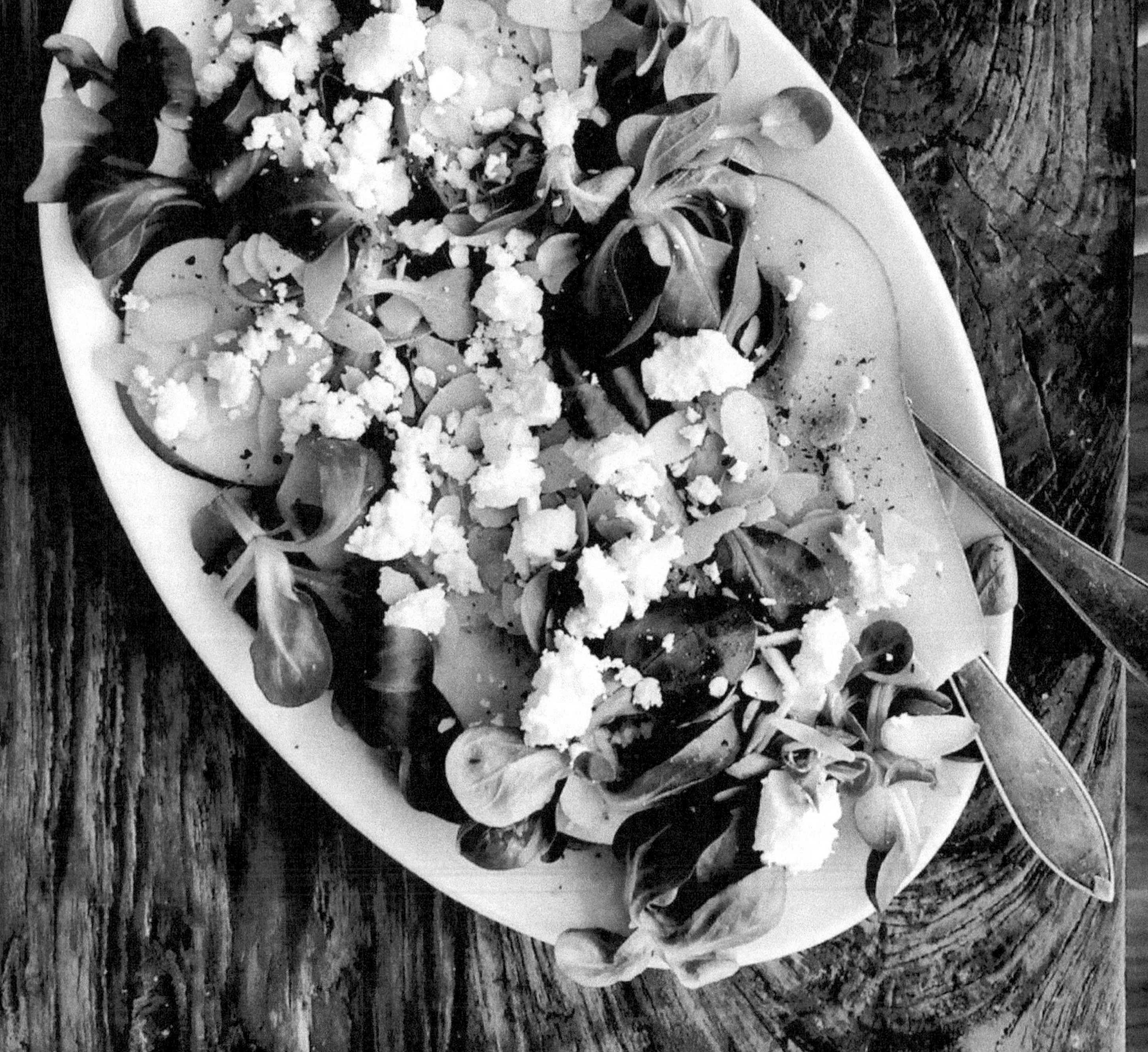

Eggplant Lasagna with Spinach and Ricotta

Prep Time: 20 Minutes | **Cook Time:** 45 Minutes | **Serves:** 4

INGREDIENTS:

- 2 large eggplants, sliced lengthwise into thin strips
- 2 cups ricotta cheese
- 1 cup fresh spinach, chopped
- 2 cups marinara sauce, low-sugar
- 1 egg
- 1 cup shredded mozzarella cheese
- 1/4 cup grated Parmesan cheese
- Salt and pepper to taste
- Olive oil for brushing

INSTRUCTIONS:

1. Preheat oven to 375°F (190°C). Brush eggplant slices with olive oil and season with salt and pepper. Arrange on baking sheets and bake for 15 minutes, until slightly tender.
2. In a bowl, mix ricotta cheese, spinach, and egg. Season with salt and pepper.
3. In a baking dish, spread a layer of marinara sauce. Add a layer of eggplant slices, followed by the ricotta mixture, and then mozzarella cheese. Repeat the layers until all ingredients are used, finishing with a layer of cheese.
4. Sprinkle Parmesan cheese on top. Bake for 30 minutes, or until the lasagna is bubbly and the top is golden.
5. Let it cool for a few minutes before serving.

NUTRITIONAL INFORMATION (PER SERVING):

Calories: 400 | Carbs: 18g | Fiber: 6g | Net Carbs: 12g
Protein: 25g | Fats: 26g

Zucchini Noodle Alfredo with Mushrooms

Prep Time: 15 Minutes | **Cook Time:** 15 Minutes | **Serves:** 4

INGREDIENTS:

- 4 medium zucchinis, spiralized into noodles
- 1 cup heavy cream
- 1 cup mushrooms, sliced
- 1/2 cup grated Parmesan cheese
- 2 tablespoons unsalted butter
- 2 cloves garlic, minced
- Salt and pepper to taste
- Fresh parsley, chopped for garnish

INSTRUCTIONS:

1. In a large skillet, melt butter over medium heat. Add garlic and mushrooms, sautéing until mushrooms are tender.
2. Add heavy cream and bring to a simmer. Stir in Parmesan cheese until melted and the sauce thickens.
3. Add zucchini noodles to the skillet, tossing gently to coat with the Alfredo sauce. Cook for 2-3 minutes until noodles are tender.
4. Season with salt and pepper to taste.
5. Serve hot, garnished with fresh parsley.

NUTRITIONAL INFORMATION (PER SERVING):

Calories: 350 | Carbs: 10g | Fiber: 2g | Net Carbs: 8g
Protein: 10g | Fats: 30g

Portobello Mushroom Steaks

Prep Time: 10 Minutes | **Cook Time:** 15 Minutes | **Serves:** 4

INGREDIENTS:

- 4 large Portobello mushroom caps
- 1/4 cup balsamic vinegar
- 1/4 cup olive oil
- 2 cloves garlic, minced
- 1 teaspoon dried thyme
- Salt and pepper to taste

INSTRUCTIONS:

1. In a bowl, whisk together balsamic vinegar, olive oil, minced garlic, thyme, salt, and pepper.
2. Place mushroom caps in a shallow dish and pour the marinade over them. Let marinate for at least 15 minutes.
3. Preheat the grill or a grill pan to medium-high heat.
4. Grill mushrooms for about 7-8 minutes per side, or until tender and grill marks appear.
5. Serve hot, optionally with additional fresh herbs or a side salad.

NUTRITIONAL INFORMATION (PER SERVING):

Calories: 150 | Carbs: 6g | Fiber: 1g | Net Carbs: 5g
Protein: 2g | Fats: 14g

Cauliflower Steaks with Chimichurri Sauce

Prep Time: 10 Minutes | **Cook Time:** 20 Minutes |
Serves: 4

INGREDIENTS:

Ingredients for Cauliflower Steaks:

- 2 large heads of cauliflower
- 2 tablespoons olive oil
- Salt and pepper to taste

Ingredients for Chimichurri Sauce:

- 1 cup fresh parsley, finely chopped
- 1/4 cup olive oil
- 2 tablespoons red wine vinegar
- 2 garlic cloves, minced
- 1/2 teaspoon red pepper flakes
- Salt to taste

INSTRUCTIONS:

1. Preheat your oven to 400°F (200°C).
2. Slice the cauliflower heads into 1-inch thick steaks and place them on a baking sheet.
3. Brush both sides of each cauliflower steak with olive oil and season with salt and pepper.
4. Roast in the oven for about 20 minutes, flipping halfway through, until tender and golden.
5. While the cauliflower is roasting, mix all the chimichurri ingredients in a bowl.
6. Serve the roasted cauliflower steaks with a generous drizzle of chimichurri sauce.

NUTRITIONAL INFORMATION (PER SERVING):

Calories: 220 | Carbs: 12g | Fiber: 5g | Net Carbs: 7g
Protein: 5g | Fats: 18g

Low-Carb "Farro" Bowl (using Cauliflower Rice)

Prep Time: 15 Minutes | **Cook Time:** 10 Minutes |
Serves: 4

INGREDIENTS:

- 1 large head of cauliflower, riced
- 2 tablespoons olive oil
- 1 cup spinach, chopped
- 1 avocado, diced
- 1/2 cup cherry tomatoes, halved
- 1/4 cup almonds, chopped
- 1/4 cup feta cheese, crumbled
- Salt and pepper to taste
- Dressing of choice (e.g., lemon vinaigrette)

INSTRUCTIONS:

1. Heat olive oil in a large skillet over medium heat.
2. Add the cauliflower rice and sauté until tender, about 5-7 minutes.
3. Assemble the bowls by dividing the cauliflower rice among them.
4. Top with spinach, avocado, cherry tomatoes, almonds, and feta cheese.
5. Drizzle with your choice of dressing and season with salt and pepper.
6. Serve immediately.

NUTRITIONAL INFORMATION (PER SERVING):

Calories: 250 | Carbs: 15g | Fiber: 7g | Net Carbs: 8g
Protein: 8g | Fats: 19g

Vegan Shepherd's Pie with Cauliflower Mash

Prep Time: 20 Minutes | **Cook Time:** 30 Minutes |
Serves: 4

INGREDIENTS:

Ingredients for the Filling:

- 2 tablespoons olive oil
- 1 onion, diced
- 2 cloves garlic, minced
- 1 cup mushrooms, chopped
- 1 cup cauliflower, finely chopped
- 1 zucchini, diced

Ingredients for the Cauliflower Mash:

- 1 large head cauliflower, cut into florets
- 2 tablespoons olive oil
- Salt and pepper to taste

- ❖ 1 bell pepper, diced
- ❖ 1 can (14 oz) diced tomatoes, drained
- ❖ 1 teaspoon thyme
- ❖ Salt and pepper to taste

INSTRUCTIONS:

1. Preheat your oven to 375°F (190°C).
2. For the cauliflower mash, steam the cauliflower florets until very tender. Blend in a food processor with olive oil, salt, and pepper until smooth.
3. Heat olive oil in a large skillet. Add onion and garlic, and sauté until translucent.
4. Add mushrooms, cauliflower, zucchini, and bell pepper. Cook until tender.
5. Stir in diced tomatoes and thyme. Season with salt and pepper. Simmer until the mixture thickens.
6. Transfer the vegetable mixture to a baking dish. Spread the cauliflower mash on top.
7. Bake for 20 minutes or until the top starts to brown.
8. Serve hot.

NUTRITIONAL INFORMATION (PER SERVING):

Calories: 220 | Carbs: 18g | Fiber: 6g | Net Carbs: 12g
Protein: 6g | Fats: 14g

Stuffed Acorn Squash with Cauliflower Rice and Nuts

Prep Time: 15 Minutes | **Cook Time:** 45 Minutes |
Serves: 4

INGREDIENTS:

- ❖ 2 acorn squash, halved and seeds removed
- ❖ 1 tablespoon olive oil
- ❖ Salt and pepper to taste
- ❖ 1/2 cup chopped nuts (e.g., pecans or walnuts)
- ❖ 1 cup cauliflower rice
- ❖ 1/4 cup diced onions
- ❖ 1 clove garlic, minced
- ❖ 1 teaspoon sage, chopped
- ❖ 1/4 cup grated Parmesan cheese

INSTRUCTIONS:

1. Preheat oven to 375°F (190°C). Brush the cut sides of the acorn squash with olive oil and season with salt and pepper. Place them cut side down on a baking sheet and roast for 30 minutes, or until tender.
2. While the squash is roasting, heat a skillet over medium heat. Add the remaining olive oil, onions, and garlic, sautéing until softened.
3. Stir in the cauliflower rice, chopped nuts, and sage. Cook until the cauliflower rice is tender, about 5-7 minutes. Season with salt and pepper.
4. Remove the roasted squash from the oven. Flip them over and fill the cavities with the cauliflower rice mixture. Sprinkle with Parmesan cheese.
5. Return to the oven and bake for an additional 15 minutes, or until the cheese is melted and golden.
6. Serve hot, garnished with more fresh sage if desired.

NUTRITIONAL INFORMATION (PER SERVING):

Calories: 220 | Carbs: 18g | Fiber: 4g | Net Carbs: 14g
Protein: 6g | Fats: 15g

Low-Carb Moussaka with Eggplant and Ground Beef

Prep Time: 30 Minutes | **Cook Time:** 1 Hour |
Serves: 4

INGREDIENTS:

- ❖ 2 large eggplants, sliced
- ❖ Salt and olive oil for eggplant
- ❖ 1 lb ground beef
- ❖ 1 can (14 oz) crushed tomatoes
- ❖ 2 cloves garlic, minced
- ❖ 1 onion, chopped
- ❖ 1 teaspoon cinnamon
- ❖ 1/2 teaspoon allspice
- ❖ Salt and pepper to taste
- ❖ For the topping: 1 cup heavy cream, 2 eggs, and 1/2 cup grated Parmesan cheese

INSTRUCTIONS:

1. Preheat your oven to 400°F (200°C). Salt the eggplant slices and let them sit for 15 minutes to draw out moisture. Pat dry, brush with olive oil, and bake for 20 minutes, flipping halfway through, until tender.
2. In a skillet, cook the ground beef, onion, and garlic until the meat is browned. Drain excess fat.

3. Stir in the crushed tomatoes, cinnamon, allspice, salt, and pepper. Simmer for 15 minutes.
4. Layer the eggplant slices and meat sauce in a baking dish.
5. Whisk together the heavy cream, eggs, and Parmesan cheese. Pour over the top layer.
6. Bake for 30 minutes, or until the topping is set and golden brown.
7. Let it cool slightly before serving.

Calories: 550 | Carbs: 18g | Fiber: 6g | Net Carbs: 12g
Protein: 30g | Fats: 40g

Spaghetti Squash Primavera

Prep Time: 15 Minutes | **Cook Time:** 45 Minutes | **Serves:** 4

INGREDIENTS:

- 1 large spaghetti squash
- 2 tablespoons olive oil
- 1 zucchini, diced
- 1 bell pepper, diced
- 1 cup cherry tomatoes, halved
- 2 cloves garlic, minced
- Salt and pepper to taste
- Fresh basil for garnish
- Grated Parmesan cheese for serving

INSTRUCTIONS:

1. Preheat your oven to 400°F (200°C). Halve the spaghetti squash and remove the seeds. Place cut side down on a baking sheet and roast for 30-40 minutes, until tender.
2. Use a fork to shred the inside of the squash into spaghetti-like strands.
3. In a skillet, heat olive oil over medium heat. Sauté zucchini and bell pepper until they start to soften, about 5-7 minutes.
4. Add cherry tomatoes and minced garlic to the skillet, and cook for an additional 2-3 minutes until the tomatoes begin to soften.
5. Season the vegetables with salt and pepper to taste. Add the shredded spaghetti squash to the skillet and toss everything together until well combined.
6. Cook for another 2-3 minutes to heat through.
7. Garnish with fresh basil leaves and serve hot, optionally sprinkled with grated Parmesan cheese.

Calories: 180 | Carbs: 17g | Fiber: 5g | Net Carbs: 12g
Protein: 4g | Fats: 12g

Cheesy Zucchini Patties

Prep Time: 15 Minutes | **Cook Time:** 10 Minutes | **Serves:** 4

INGREDIENTS:

- 2 medium zucchinis, grated
- 1/2 cup almond flour
- 1/2 cup grated Parmesan cheese
- 1 egg, beaten
- 2 cloves garlic, minced
- Salt and pepper to taste
- 2 tablespoons olive oil for frying

INSTRUCTIONS:

1. Place the grated zucchini in a colander, sprinkle with salt, and let it sit for 10 minutes to draw out moisture. Squeeze out the excess water using a clean kitchen towel.
2. In a bowl, mix the drained zucchini with almond flour, Parmesan cheese, beaten egg, minced garlic, and season with salt and pepper.
3. Heat olive oil in a skillet over medium heat. Form the zucchini mixture into patties and fry for about 5 minutes on each side, or until golden brown and crispy.
4. Serve hot, optionally with a side of low-carb sour cream or yogurt.

Calories: 200 | Carbs: 6g | Fiber: 2g | Net Carbs: 4g
Protein: 10g | Fats: 15g

Caprese Stuffed Avocado

Prep Time: 10 Minutes | **Cook Time:** 0 Minute | **Serves:** 4

INGREDIENTS:

- 2 large avocados, halved and pitted
- 1 cup cherry tomatoes, halved
- 1/2 cup mozzarella balls, halved
- 1/4 cup fresh basil leaves, chopped

❖ 1 Balsamic glaze for drizzling

❖ Salt and pepper to taste

❖ Extra virgin olive oil for drizzling

INSTRUCTIONS:

1. Scoop out some of the avocado flesh to create more space for the filling, leaving a thick border.
2. In a bowl, toss together cherry tomatoes, mozzarella balls, and chopped basil. Season with salt and pepper.
3. Fill the avocado halves with the tomato and mozzarella mixture.
4. Drizzle with balsamic glaze and olive oil before serving.
5. Serve immediately as a fresh and healthy appetizer or light meal.

NUTRITIONAL INFORMATION (PER SERVING):

Calories: 250 | Carbs: 12g | Fiber: 7g | Net Carbs: 5g
Protein: 8g | Fats: 20g

Broccoli and Cheddar Stuffed Peppers

Prep Time: 15 Minutes | **Cook Time:** 25 Minutes |
Serves: 4

INGREDIENTS:

❖ 4 bell peppers, halved and seeded

❖ 2 cups broccoli florets, finely chopped

❖ 1 cup cooked chicken, shredded (optional for added protein)

❖ 1/4 cup cream cheese, softened

❖ 1/2 cup sour cream

❖ Salt and pepper to taste

❖ Paprika for sprinkling

❖ 1 cup cheddar cheese, shredded

INSTRUCTIONS:

1. Preheat your oven to 375°F (190°C). Place the bell pepper halves in a baking dish.
2. In a bowl, mix together the chopped broccoli, shredded chicken (if using), cheddar cheese, cream cheese, and sour cream. Season with salt and pepper.
3. Stuff the bell pepper halves with the broccoli and cheese mixture. Sprinkle the tops with paprika.
4. Bake in the preheated oven for 25 minutes, or until the peppers are tender and the filling is bubbly and golden.

5. Serve hot as a nutritious and satisfying main dish or side.

NUTRITIONAL INFORMATION (PER SERVING):

Calories: 300 | Carbs: 10g | Fiber: 3g | Net Carbs: 7g
Protein: 12g | Fats: 24g

Stuffed Acorn Squash

Prep Time: 20 Minutes | **Cook Time:** 50 Minutes |
Serves: 4

INGREDIENTS:

❖ 2 acorn squash, halved and seeds removed

❖ 1 tablespoon olive oil

❖ Salt and pepper to taste

❖ 1 cup cauliflower rice

❖ 1/2 pound ground turkey or beef (optional for a non-vegetarian version)

❖ 1 small onion, diced

❖ 1 clove garlic, minced

❖ 1 teaspoon sage, chopped

❖ 1/2 cup mushrooms, chopped

❖ 1/4 cup pecans, chopped

❖ 1/4 cup Parmesan cheese, grated

INSTRUCTIONS:

1. Preheat your oven to 375°F (190°C). Brush the inside of each squash half with olive oil and season with salt and pepper. Place on a baking sheet, cut side down, and roast for about 40 minutes, until tender.
2. In a skillet, heat a bit more olive oil over medium heat. Sauté onion, garlic, and mushrooms until softened. Add ground meat if using, and cook until browned.
3. Stir in the cauliflower rice and sage. Cook until the cauliflower is tender. Season with salt and pepper.
4. Mix in the pecans and remove from heat.
5. Fill the roasted squash halves with the cauliflower mixture. Sprinkle with Parmesan cheese.
6. Return to the oven for about 10 minutes, until the filling is heated through and the cheese is melted.
7. Serve warm.

NUTRITIONAL INFORMATION (PER SERVING):

Calories: 300 | Carbs: 20g | Fiber: 5g | Net Carbs: 15g
Protein: 15g | Fats: 18g

Vegetable Korma with Cauliflower Rice

Prep Time: 15 Minutes | **Cook Time:** 25 Minutes | **Serves:** 4

INGREDIENTS:

* 1 head cauliflower, riced
* 2 tablespoons coconut oil
* 1 onion, diced
* 1 tablespoon ginger, minced
* 1 tablespoon curry powder
* 1/2 cup coconut milk
* 1 cup mixed vegetables (carrots, peas, bell peppers), chopped
* Salt and pepper to taste
* Fresh cilantro for garnish

INSTRUCTIONS:

1. In a skillet, heat the coconut oil over medium heat. Add the onion and ginger, sautéing until the onion is translucent.
2. Stir in the curry powder, cooking for another minute until fragrant.
3. Add the mixed vegetables and coconut milk. Simmer for about 15 minutes, until the vegetables are tender.
4. In another pan, sauté the cauliflower rice in a bit of coconut oil until tender, about 5-7 minutes.
5. Serve the vegetable korma over the cauliflower rice, garnished with fresh cilantro.

NUTRITIONAL INFORMATION (PER SERVING):

Calories: 180 | Carbs: 15g | Fiber: 5g | Net Carbs: 10g
Protein: 4g | Fats: 12g

Creamy Spinach and Artichoke Casserole

Prep Time: 15 Minutes | **Cook Time:** 30 Minutes | **Serves:** 4

INGREDIENTS:

* 2 cups spinach, chopped
* 1 can (14 oz) artichoke hearts, drained and chopped
* 1 cup cream cheese, softened
* 1/2 cup sour cream
* 1/2 cup grated Parmesan cheese
* 2 cloves garlic, minced
* Salt and pepper to taste

INSTRUCTIONS:

1. Preheat your oven to 350°F (175°C).
2. In a large bowl, mix together the cream cheese, sour cream, Parmesan cheese, and minced garlic until smooth.
3. Stir in the chopped spinach and artichoke hearts. Season with salt and pepper.
4. Transfer the mixture to a baking dish and spread evenly.
5. Bake for about 30 minutes, until the top is golden and bubbly.
6. Serve warm as a side dish or a dip with low-carb crackers or vegetable sticks.

NUTRITIONAL INFORMATION (PER SERVING):

Calories: 350 | Carbs: 10g | Fiber: 3g | Net Carbs: 7g
Protein: 10g | Fats: 30g

Shakshuka with Feta

Prep Time: 10 Minutes | **Cook Time:** 20 Minutes | **Serves:** 4

INGREDIENTS:

* 1 tablespoon olive oil
* 1 onion, diced
* 1 bell pepper, diced
* 2 cloves garlic, minced
* 1 can (14 oz) diced tomatoes
* 1 teaspoon paprika
* 1/2 teaspoon cumin
* Salt and pepper to taste
* 4 large eggs
* 1/2 cup feta cheese, crumbled
* Fresh parsley, chopped for garnish

INSTRUCTIONS:

1. Heat olive oil in a large skillet over medium heat. Add onion and bell pepper, and cook until softened.
2. Add minced garlic, diced tomatoes, paprika, and cumin. Season with salt and pepper. Simmer for 10 minutes until the sauce thickens slightly.
3. Make four wells in the sauce and crack an egg into each well. Cover the skillet and cook until eggs are set to your liking.
4. Sprinkle crumbled feta cheese and chopped parsley over the top.
5. Serve hot directly from the skillet.

Calories: 200 | Carbs: 10g | Fiber: 2g | Net Carbs: 8g

Protein: 12g | Fats: 14g

Keto Veggie Burger with Portobello Bun

Prep Time: 15 Minutes | **Cook Time:** 15 Minutes | **Serves:** 4

INGREDIENTS:

- 4 large Portobello mushroom caps
- 1 tablespoon olive oil
- 4 keto-friendly veggie burger patties (homemade or store-bought)
- 1 avocado, sliced
- 1 tomato, sliced
- Lettuce leaves
- Salt and pepper to taste
- Mustard and sugar-free ketchup for serving (optional)

INSTRUCTIONS:

1. Brush Portobello caps with olive oil and season with salt and pepper. Grill or bake at 400°F (200°C) for about 5-7 minutes per side, until tender.
2. Grill or cook the veggie burger patties according to package instructions or your recipe.
3. Assemble the burgers using Portobello mushrooms as buns, with a veggie patty, avocado slices, tomato slices, and lettuce leaves in between.
4. Serve with mustard and sugar-free ketchup if desired.

NUTRITIONAL INFORMATION (PER SERVING):

Calories: 250 | Carbs: 12g | Fiber: 6g | Net Carbs: 6g

Protein: 20g | Fats: 16g

Low-Carb Ratatouille with Tofu

Prep Time: 20 Minutes | **Cook Time:** 40 Minutes | **Serves:** 4

INGREDIENTS:

- 2 tablespoons olive oil, divided
- 1 small eggplant, sliced
- 1 block (14 oz) firm tofu, drained and cubed
- 1 yellow squash, sliced
- 1 red bell pepper, sliced
- 1 can (14 oz) crushed tomatoes
- 2 zucchinis, sliced
- 2 cloves garlic, minced
- 1 teaspoon dried thyme
- Salt and pepper to taste
- Fresh basil for garnish

INSTRUCTIONS:

1. Press tofu to remove excess water, then cube.
2. Heat 1 tablespoon olive oil in a skillet over medium heat. Sauté tofu until golden brown. Set aside.
3. In the same skillet, add the remaining olive oil. Sauté garlic for 1 minute. Add crushed tomatoes and thyme. Season with salt and pepper. Simmer for 5 minutes to create a sauce.
4. In a baking dish, layer eggplant, zucchini, yellow squash, and red bell pepper slices. Pour the tomato sauce over the vegetables.
5. Bake in a preheated oven at 375°F (190°C) for 35 minutes, until vegetables are tender.
6. Serve the ratatouille topped with sautéed tofu and garnished with fresh basil.

NUTRITIONAL INFORMATION (PER SERVING):

Calories: 220 | Carbs: 18g | Fiber: 6g | Net Carbs: 12g

Protein: 15g | Fats: 12g

Grilled Halloumi and Vegetable Skewers

Prep Time: 15 Minutes | **Cook Time:** 10 Minutes | **Serves:** 4

INGREDIENTS:

- 8 oz halloumi cheese, cut into cubes
- 1 zucchini, cut into chunks
- 1 red bell pepper, cut into chunks
- 1 yellow bell pepper, cut into chunks
- 8 cherry tomatoes
- 1/4 cup olive oil
- 2 tablespoons lemon juice
- 1 teaspoon dried oregano
- Salt and pepper to taste
- Fresh parsley, chopped for garnish

INSTRUCTIONS:

1. In a bowl, whisk together olive oil, lemon juice, oregano, salt, and pepper to make the marinade.
2. Thread halloumi, zucchini, bell peppers, and cherry tomatoes onto skewers.
3. Brush the skewers with the marinade and let them sit for at least 30 minutes.
4. Preheat the grill to medium-high heat. Grill the skewers for about 10 minutes, turning occasionally, until the vegetables are tender and the halloumi has grill marks.
5. Garnish with fresh parsley before serving.

NUTRITIONAL INFORMATION (PER SERVING):

Calories: 280 | Carbs: 6g | Fiber: 2g | Net Carbs: 4g
Protein: 14g | Fats: 22g

Palak Paneer with Tofu

Prep Time: 20 Minutes | **Cook Time:** 30 Minutes |
Serves: 4

INGREDIENTS:

- 14 oz firm tofu, pressed and cubed (as a substitute for paneer)
- 10 oz fresh spinach, blanched and pureed
- 2 tablespoons olive oil
- 1 onion, finely chopped
- 1 teaspoon minced ginger
- 1 teaspoon minced garlic
- 1 teaspoon garam masala
- 1/2 teaspoon turmeric
- 1/2 teaspoon cumin
- 1/2 cup tomato puree
- Salt to taste
- 1/4 cup heavy cream (optional for creaminess)
- Fresh cilantro for garnish

INSTRUCTIONS:

1. Heat 1 tablespoon olive oil in a pan and fry the tofu cubes until golden brown. Set aside.
2. In the same pan, heat the remaining olive oil and sauté onion, ginger, and garlic until the onion is translucent.
3. Add garam masala, turmeric, and cumin, and cook for another minute.
4. Stir in the tomato puree and cook for 5 minutes.
5. Add the pureed spinach and cooked tofu to the pan. Season with salt and simmer for 10 minutes. If using, stir in heavy cream for the last 2 minutes.

6. Garnish with fresh cilantro and serve with cauliflower rice.

NUTRITIONAL INFORMATION (PER SERVING):

Calories: 200 | Carbs: 8g | Fiber: 3g | Net Carbs: 5g
Protein: 12g | Fats: 14g

Stuffed Cabbage Rolls with Cauliflower

Prep Time: 30 Minutes | **Cook Time:** 1 Hour |
Serves: 4

INGREDIENTS:

- 8 large cabbage leaves
- 1 lb ground turkey or beef
- 2 cups cauliflower rice
- 1 small onion, diced
- 1 can (14 oz) diced tomatoes
- 2 cloves garlic, minced
- 1 teaspoon paprika
- Salt and pepper to taste
- 1/2 cup low-sugar tomato sauce

INSTRUCTIONS:

1. Blanch the cabbage leaves in boiling water for 2 minutes. Drain and set aside.
2. In a skillet, cook the ground meat, onion, and garlic until the meat is browned. Drain excess fat.
3. Mix in the cauliflower rice, diced tomatoes, paprika, salt, and pepper. Cook for 5 minutes.
4. Place some of the meat mixture in the center of each cabbage leaf. Fold in the sides and roll up the leaf to enclose the filling.
5. Place the cabbage rolls seam side down in a baking dish. Pour the tomato sauce over the rolls.
6. Cover with foil and bake at 350°F (175°C) for about 1 hour.
7. Serve hot, garnished with fresh herbs if desired.

NUTRITIONAL INFORMATION (PER SERVING):

Calories: 250 | Carbs: 15g | Fiber: 5g | Net Carbs: 11g
Protein: 28g | Fats: 8g

Cheesy Zucchini Boats

Prep Time: 15 Minutes | **Cook Time:** 20 Minutes |
Serves: 4

INGREDIENTS:

- 4 medium zucchinis, halved lengthwise
- 1 cup marinara sauce, low-sugar
- 1 cup shredded mozzarella cheese
- Olive oil for brushing
- 1/2 cup grated Parmesan cheese
- 1/4 cup fresh basil, chopped
- Salt and pepper to taste

INSTRUCTIONS:

1. Preheat your oven to 375°F (190°C). Scoop out the center of each zucchini half to create a 'boat'.
2. Brush the zucchini boats lightly with olive oil and season with salt and pepper. Place them on a baking sheet.
3. Spoon marinara sauce into each zucchini boat. Sprinkle mozzarella and Parmesan cheeses on top.
4. Bake for 20 minutes, or until the cheese is melted and bubbly, and the zucchini is tender.
5. Garnish with fresh basil before serving.

NUTRITIONAL INFORMATION (PER SERVING):

Calories: 200 | Carbs: 10g | Fiber: 2g | Net Carbs: 8g
Protein: 15g | Fats: 12g

Crispy Eggplant Rounds

Prep Time: 20 Minutes | **Cook Time:** 30 Minutes |
Serves: 4

INGREDIENTS:

- 1 large eggplant, sliced into 1/2-inch rounds
- Salt for drawing out moisture
- 1/2 cup almond flour
- 2 eggs, beaten
- 1 cup grated Parmesan cheese
- 1 teaspoon Italian seasoning
- Olive oil for baking

INSTRUCTIONS:

1. Salt both sides of the eggplant slices and let them sit for about 15 minutes to draw out moisture. Pat dry with paper towels.
2. Preheat the oven to 400°F (200°C) and grease a baking sheet with olive oil.
3. Mix almond flour, Parmesan cheese, and Italian seasoning in one bowl. Place beaten eggs in another bowl.
4. Dip each eggplant round first in the egg, then in the almond flour mixture, ensuring it's well-coated.
5. Place the coated eggplant rounds on the prepared baking sheet and bake for 30 minutes, flipping halfway through, until golden and crispy.
6. Serve hot, with a side of low-sugar marinara sauce for dipping if desired.

NUTRITIONAL INFORMATION (PER SERVING):

Calories: 250 | Carbs: 15g | Fiber: 6g | Net Carbs: 9g
Protein: 20g | Fats: 15g

Vegan Cauliflower Tacos

Prep Time: 15 Minutes | **Cook Time:** 25 Minutes |
Serves: 4

INGREDIENTS:

- 1 head cauliflower, cut into small florets
- 1 tablespoon olive oil
- 1 teaspoon chili powder
- 1/2 teaspoon cumin
- 1/2 teaspoon paprika
- Salt and pepper to taste
- 8 low-carb tortillas
- 1 avocado, sliced
- 1/4 cup red cabbage, shredded
- 1/4 cup fresh cilantro, chopped
- Lime wedges for serving

INSTRUCTIONS:

1. Preheat your oven to 425°F (220°C). Toss cauliflower florets with olive oil, chili powder, cumin, paprika, salt, and pepper.
2. Spread the seasoned cauliflower on a baking sheet and roast for 25 minutes, or until tender and slightly caramelized.
3. Warm the low-carb tortillas according to package instructions.
4. Assemble the tacos by placing roasted cauliflower in each tortilla, topped with avocado slices, shredded cabbage, and fresh cilantro.
5. Serve with lime wedges on the side for squeezing over the tacos.

NUTRITIONAL INFORMATION (PER SERVING):

Calories: 300 | Carbs: 25g | Fiber: 15g | Net Carbs: 10g
Protein: 10g | Fats: 20g

Bell Pepper and Eggplant Stir-Fry

Prep Time: 15 Minutes | **Cook Time:** 15 Minutes | **Serves:** 4

INGREDIENTS:

- 1 large eggplant, cubed
- 2 bell peppers (any color), sliced
- 1 onion, sliced
- 2 tablespoons olive oil
- 2 cloves garlic, minced
- 2 tablespoons soy sauce or tamari (gluten-free)
- 1 teaspoon ginger, grated
- Salt and pepper to taste
- Sesame seeds for garnish

INSTRUCTIONS:

1. Heat olive oil in a large skillet or wok over medium-high heat. Add eggplant, bell peppers, and onion, and stir-fry until they start to soften, about 5-7 minutes.
2. Add minced garlic and grated ginger to the skillet, cooking for another minute until fragrant.
3. Stir in soy sauce or tamari, and continue to cook for another 5 minutes, until the vegetables are fully cooked and coated in the sauce.
4. Season with salt and pepper to taste.
5. Serve hot, garnished with sesame seeds.

NUTRITIONAL INFORMATION (PER SERVING):

Calories: 160 | Carbs: 15g | Fiber: 5g | Net Carbs: 10g
Protein: 3g | Fats: 10g

Asparagus and Leek Quiche with Almond Flour Crust

Prep Time: 20 Minutes | **Cook Time:** 35 Minutes | **Serves:** 6

INGREDIENTS:

Ingredients for Filling:

Ingredients for Crust:

- 1 tablespoon olive oil
- 4 large eggs
- 1 leek, white and light green parts only, thinly sliced
- 1 cup asparagus, chopped into 1-inch pieces
- 1 1/2 cups almond flour
- 1/4 cup unsalted butter, melted
- 1/4 teaspoon salt

INSTRUCTIONS:

1. Preheat your oven to 350°F (175°C). Mix almond flour, melted butter, and salt in a bowl until a dough forms. Press the dough into a 9-inch pie dish to form the crust. Bake for 10 minutes until slightly golden. Remove from the oven and set aside.
2. Heat olive oil in a skillet over medium heat. Add leek and asparagus, sautéing until softened, about 5-7 minutes.
3. In a bowl, whisk together eggs, heavy cream, and Parmesan cheese. Season with salt and pepper.
4. Spread the sautéed leek and asparagus evenly over the pre-baked crust. Pour the egg mixture over the vegetables.
5. Bake for 25-30 minutes, or until the quiche is set and the top is lightly golden.
6. Let it cool for a few minutes before slicing and serving.

NUTRITIONAL INFORMATION (PER SERVING):

Calories: 380 | Carbs: 12g | Fiber: 4g | Net Carbs: 8g
Protein: 14g | Fats: 32g

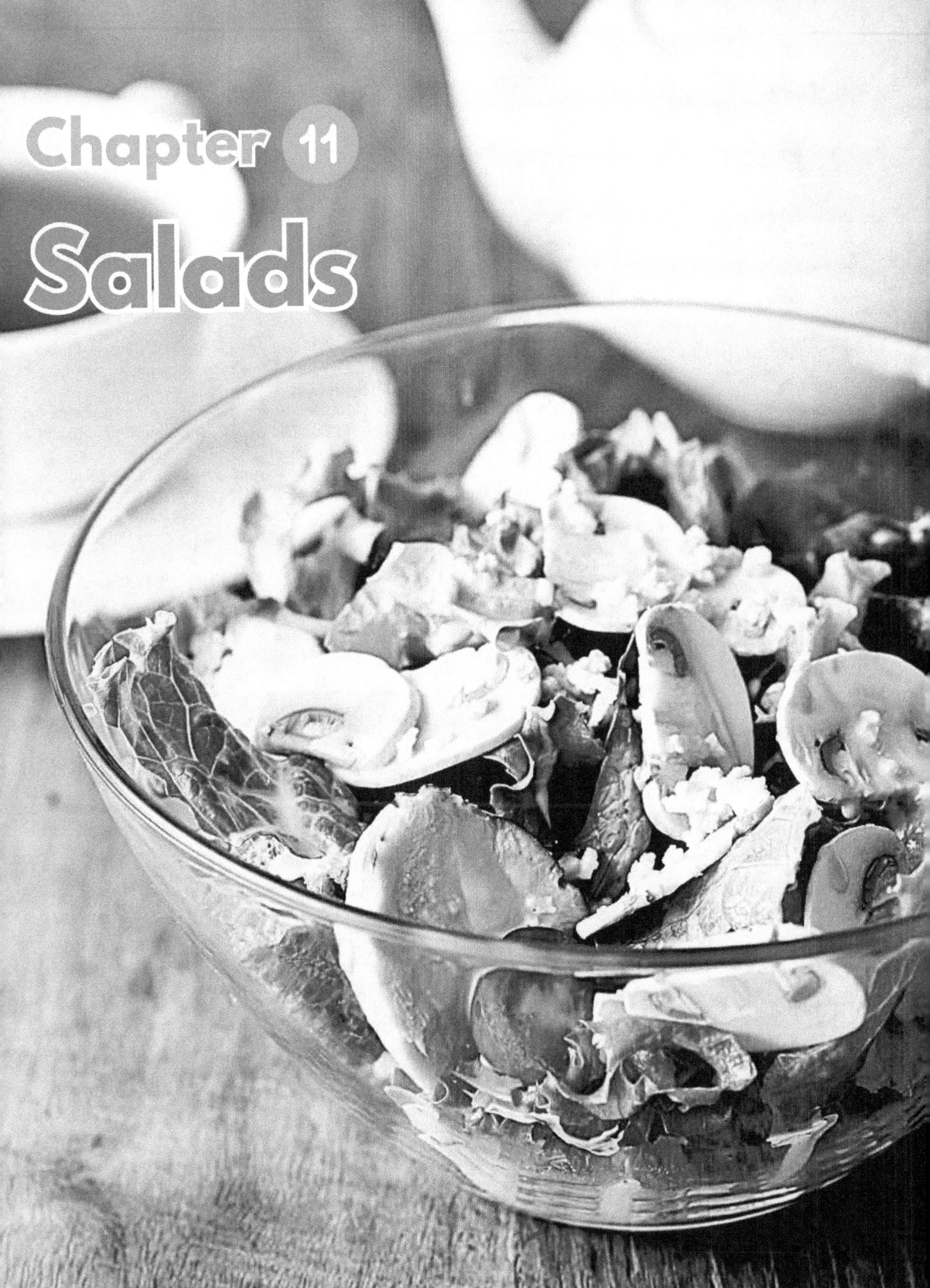

Chapter 11
Salads

Avocado and Egg Breakfast Salad

Prep Time: 10 Minutes | **Cook Time:** 5 Minutes | **Serves:** 2

INGREDIENTS:

- 2 large eggs, boiled to your preference
- 1 large avocado, cubed
- 2 cups mixed salad greens
- 1/2 cup cherry tomatoes, halved
- 2 tablespoons olive oil
- 1 tablespoon lemon juice
- Salt and pepper to taste
- Fresh herbs (such as parsley or chives) for garnish

INSTRUCTIONS:

1. Peel and slice or chop the boiled eggs to your preference.
2. In a large bowl, combine the mixed salad greens, cherry tomatoes, and cubed avocado.
3. In a small bowl, whisk together olive oil and lemon juice. Season with salt and pepper.
4. Drizzle the dressing over the salad and gently toss to combine.
5. Top the salad with the boiled eggs and garnish with fresh herbs.
6. Serve immediately as a nutritious and filling breakfast or brunch dish.

NUTRITIONAL INFORMATION (PER SERVING):

Calories: 350 | Carbs: 12g | Fiber: 7g | Net Carbs: 5g
Protein: 10g | Fats: 30g

Spinach and Goat Cheese Salad with Raspberry Vinaigrette

Prep Time: 15 Minutes | **Cook Time:** 0 Minute | **Serves:** 4

INGREDIENTS:

Ingredients for Salad:

- 1/2 cup goat cheese, crumbled

Ingredients for Raspberry Vinaigrette:

- 1/4 cup fresh raspberries

- 6 cups fresh spinach leaves, washed and dried
- 1/4 cup walnuts, toasted and chopped
- 1/2 cup fresh raspberries
- 2 tablespoons olive oil
- 1 tablespoon balsamic vinegar
- 1 teaspoon Dijon mustard
- Salt and pepper to taste

INSTRUCTIONS:

1. In a large salad bowl, combine spinach leaves, crumbled goat cheese, toasted walnuts, and fresh raspberries.
2. To make the vinaigrette, blend 1/4 cup raspberries, olive oil, balsamic vinegar, Dijon mustard, salt, and pepper until smooth.
3. Drizzle the raspberry vinaigrette over the salad and gently toss to coat.
4. Serve immediately, enjoying the blend of creamy goat cheese, tangy raspberries, and crunchy walnuts.

NUTRITIONAL INFORMATION (PER SERVING):

Calories: 200 | Carbs: 6g | Fiber: 3g | Net Carbs: 3g
Protein: 6g | Fats: 16g

Shrimp and Avocado Caesar Salad

Prep Time: 20 Minutes | **Cook Time:** 5 Minutes | **Serves:** 4

INGREDIENTS:

- 1 pound cooked shrimp, peeled and deveined
- 6 cups romaine lettuce, chopped
- 1/2 cup Parmesan cheese, shaved
- 2 large avocados, diced
- Caesar dressing, low-carb and sugar-free
- Salt and pepper to taste
- Lemon wedges for serving

INSTRUCTIONS:

1. In a large salad bowl, toss the chopped romaine lettuce with Caesar dressing until evenly coated. Season with salt and pepper to taste.
2. Add the cooked shrimp and diced avocados to the salad. Gently toss to combine.
3. Top the salad with shaved Parmesan cheese.

4. Serve the salad with lemon wedges on the side for an
    added zesty flavor.

NUTRITIONAL INFORMATION (PER SERVING):

Calories: 300 | Carbs: 8g | Fiber: 5g | Net Carbs: 3g
Protein: 25g | Fats: 18g

Mediterranean Tuna Salad

Prep Time: 15 Minutes | **Cook Time:** 0 Minutes
Serves: 4

INGREDIENTS:

- 2 cans (5 oz each) tuna in olive oil, drained
- 1 cup cherry tomatoes, halved
- 1 cucumber, diced
- 1/2 red onion, thinly sliced
- 1/4 cup Kalamata olives, pitted and halved
- 1/4 cup feta cheese, crumbled
- 2 tablespoons extra virgin olive oil
- 1 tablespoon lemon juice
- 1 teaspoon dried oregano
- Salt and pepper to taste

INSTRUCTIONS:

1. In a large mixing bowl, combine the drained tuna, halved cherry tomatoes, diced cucumber, sliced red onion, and Kalamata olives.
2. In a small bowl, whisk together the extra virgin olive oil, lemon juice, dried oregano, salt, and pepper to create the dressing.
3. Pour the dressing over the tuna salad and gently toss to combine all the ingredients.
4. Sprinkle crumbled feta cheese over the top of the salad.
5. Serve the Mediterranean Tuna Salad chilled or at room temperature, enjoying the fresh, vibrant flavors.

NUTRITIONAL INFORMATION (PER SERVING):

Calories: 250 | Carbs: 6g | Fiber: 2g | Net Carbs: 4g
Protein: 20g | Fats: 16g

Kale and Roasted Almond Salad

Prep Time: 15 Minutes | **Cook Time:** 10 Minutes
Serves: 4

INGREDIENTS:

- 6 cups kale, stems removed and leaves chopped
- 1/2 cup almonds, roughly chopped
- 1/4 cup Parmesan cheese, shaved
- 1/4 cup olive oil
- 2 tablespoons lemon juice
- 1 clove garlic, minced
- Salt and pepper to taste

INSTRUCTIONS:

1. Preheat the oven to 350°F (175°C). Spread the chopped almonds on a baking sheet and roast for about 10 minutes, or until golden and fragrant. Let cool.
2. In a large salad bowl, combine the chopped kale and roasted almonds.
3. In a small bowl, whisk together olive oil, lemon juice, minced garlic, salt, and pepper to create the dressing.
4. Pour the dressing over the kale and almond mixture, and toss well to coat the leaves evenly.
5. Top the salad with shaved Parmesan cheese before serving.

NUTRITIONAL INFORMATION (PER SERVING):

Calories: 250 | Carbs: 10g | Fiber: 3g | Net Carbs: 7g
Protein: 8g | Fats: 20g

Cobb Salad with Turkey Bacon

Prep Time: 20 Minutes | **Cook Time:** 10 Minutes
Serves: 4

INGREDIENTS:

- 8 slices turkey bacon, cooked and crumbled
- 6 cups mixed salad greens
- 2 hard-boiled eggs, diced
- 1 avocado, diced
- 1 cup cherry tomatoes, halved
- 1/2 cup blue cheese, crumbled
- 1/4 cup red onion, thinly sliced
- Ranch or blue cheese dressing, low-carb

1. Cook the turkey bacon in a skillet over medium heat until crispy. Let cool, then crumble.
2. Arrange mixed salad greens in a large salad bowl or on individual plates.
3. Top the greens with rows of diced hard-boiled eggs, diced avocado, halved cherry tomatoes, crumbled blue cheese, sliced red onion, and crumbled turkey bacon.
4. Serve the salad with low-carb ranch or blue cheese dressing on the side.

NUTRITIONAL INFORMATION (PER SERVING):

Calories: 300 | Carbs: 10g | Fiber: 5g | Net Carbs: 5g

Protein: 20g | Fats: 20g

Broccoli and Bacon Salad with Cheddar

Prep Time: 15 Minutes | **Cook Time:** 10 Minutes | **Serves:** 4

INGREDIENTS:

- 4 cups broccoli florets
- 6 slices bacon, cooked and crumbled
- 1/2 cup sharp cheddar cheese, shredded
- 1/4 cup red onion, finely chopped
- 1/2 cup mayonnaise, low-carb
- 2 tablespoons apple cider vinegar
- 1 tablespoon erythritol or other low-carb sweetener
- Salt and pepper to taste

INSTRUCTIONS:

1. Steam the broccoli florets for about 3-4 minutes until just tender. Rinse under cold water to stop the cooking process and drain well.
2. In a large mixing bowl, combine the steamed broccoli, crumbled bacon, shredded cheddar cheese, and chopped red onion.
3. In a small bowl, whisk together mayonnaise, apple cider vinegar, erythritol, salt, and pepper to create the dressing.
4. Pour the dressing over the broccoli mixture and toss to coat evenly.
5. Refrigerate the salad for at least 30 minutes before serving to allow the flavors to meld.

NUTRITIONAL INFORMATION (PER SERVING):

Calories: 350 | Carbs: 8g | Fiber: 2g | Net Carbs: 6g

Protein: 12g | Fats: 30g

Herbed Tomato Salad

Prep Time: 10 Minutes | **Cook Time:** 0 Minutes | **Serves:** 4

INGREDIENTS:

- 4 large ripe tomatoes, sliced
- 1/4 cup fresh basil leaves, chopped
- 1/4 cup fresh parsley, chopped
- 2 tablespoons olive oil
- 1 tablespoon balsamic vinegar
- Salt and pepper to taste
- 1/4 cup feta cheese, crumbled (optional)

INSTRUCTIONS:

1. Arrange the sliced tomatoes on a serving platter.
2. Sprinkle the chopped basil and parsley evenly over the tomatoes.
3. Drizzle olive oil and balsamic vinegar over the top.
4. Season with salt and pepper to taste.
5. If using, sprinkle crumbled feta cheese over the salad before serving.
6. Serve immediately or chill for a short time to allow flavors to meld.

NUTRITIONAL INFORMATION (PER SERVING):

Calories: 90 | Carbs: 6g | Fiber: 2g | Net Carbs: 4g

Protein: 2g | Fats: 7g

Asian Chicken Salad with Ginger Sesame Dressing

Prep Time: 20 Minutes | **Cook Time:** 15 Minutes | **Serves:** 4

INGREDIENTS:

Ingredients for Salad:
- 2 cups cooked chicken, shredded

Ingredients for Ginger Sesame Dressing:
- 1 tablespoon vinegar

- ❖ 4 cups mixed salad greens
- ❖ 1 cup red cabbage, shredded
- ❖ 1 bell pepper, thinly sliced
- ❖ 1/2 cup cucumber, sliced
- ❖ 1/4 cup green onions, chopped
- ❖ 1/4 cup almonds, slivered
- ❖ 2 tablespoons sesame oil
- ❖ 2 tablespoons soy sauce or tamari for gluten-free option
- ❖ 1 tablespoon ginger, grated
- ❖ 1 clove garlic, minced
- ❖ 1 teaspoon erythritol or other low-carb sweetener

1. In a large salad bowl, combine the salad greens, red cabbage, bell pepper, cucumber, green onions, and cooked chicken.
2. In a small bowl, whisk together the sesame oil, soy sauce, vinegar, grated ginger, minced garlic, and erythritol to make the dressing.
3. Pour the dressing over the salad and toss to combine.
4. Sprinkle slivered almonds over the top.
5. Serve the salad immediately, ensuring the vegetables stay crisp and fresh.

NUTRITIONAL INFORMATION (PER SERVING):

Calories: 250 | Carbs: 8g | Fiber: 3g | Net Carbs: 5g

Protein: 20g | Fats: 16g

Cucumber and Dill Salad with Feta

Prep Time: 10 Minutes | **Cook Time:** 0 Minutes | **Serves:** 4

INGREDIENTS:

- ❖ 2 large cucumbers, thinly sliced
- ❖ 1/4 cup red onion, thinly sliced
- ❖ 1/4 cup fresh dill, chopped
- ❖ 1/4 cup feta cheese, crumbled
- ❖ 2 tablespoons olive oil
- ❖ 1 tablespoon lemon juice
- ❖ Salt and pepper to taste

INSTRUCTIONS:

1. In a large salad bowl, combine the thinly sliced cucumbers, red onion, and chopped dill.
2. In a small bowl, whisk together the olive oil and lemon juice. Season with salt and pepper.
3. Pour the dressing over the cucumber mixture and toss gently to coat.
4. Sprinkle crumbled feta cheese over the salad.
5. Serve immediately, or chill in the refrigerator for 30 minutes before serving for enhanced flavors.

NUTRITIONAL INFORMATION (PER SERVING):

Calories: 120 | Carbs: 5g | Fiber: 1g | Net Carbs: 4g

Protein: 3g | Fats: 10g

Grilled Salmon Salad with Citrus Dressing

Prep Time: 15 Minutes | **Cook Time:** 10 Minutes | **Serves:** 4

INGREDIENTS:

Ingredients for Salad:

- ❖ 4 salmon fillets (4 oz each)
- ❖ 8 cups mixed greens
- ❖ 1 avocado, sliced
- ❖ 1/2 red onion, thinly sliced
- ❖ 1/4 cup almond slices, toasted

Ingredients for Citrus Dressing:

- ❖ 1/4 cup olive oil
- ❖ 2 tablespoons orange juice, freshly squeezed
- ❖ 1 tablespoon lemon juice, freshly squeezed
- ❖ 1 teaspoon Dijon mustard
- ❖ Salt and pepper to taste

INSTRUCTIONS:

1. Preheat the grill to medium-high heat. Grill salmon fillets for about 5 minutes on each side, or until cooked through and easily flaked with a fork.
2. In a large salad bowl, combine mixed greens, sliced avocado, and red onion.
3. For the dressing, whisk together olive oil, orange juice, lemon juice, Dijon mustard, salt, and pepper in a small bowl.
4. Drizzle the citrus dressing over the salad and toss to combine.
5. Divide the salad among plates, top each with a grilled salmon fillet and sprinkle with toasted almond slices.
6. Serve immediately.

Edamame and Walnut Salad

Prep Time: 10 Minutes | **Cook Time:** 5 Minutes | **Serves:** 4

INGREDIENTS:

- 2 cups shelled edamame, cooked and cooled
- 1 cup walnuts, roughly chopped
- 2 cups mixed salad greens
- 1/4 cup feta cheese, crumbled
- 2 tablespoons olive oil
- 1 tablespoon white wine vinegar
- Salt and pepper to taste

INSTRUCTIONS:

1. In a large salad bowl, combine the cooked edamame, chopped walnuts, and mixed salad greens.
2. Add crumbled feta cheese to the bowl.
3. In a small bowl, whisk together olive oil and white wine vinegar. Season with salt and pepper.
4. Drizzle the dressing over the salad and toss gently to combine all ingredients.
5. Serve the salad chilled or at room temperature.

NUTRITIONAL INFORMATION (PER SERVING):

Calories: 320 | Carbs: 10g | Fiber: 5g | Net Carbs: 5g
Protein: 15g | Fats: 25g

Arugula, Pear, and Blue Cheese Salad

Prep Time: 10 Minutes | **Cook Time:** 0 Minute | **Serves:** 4

INGREDIENTS:

- 6 cups arugula
- 1 ripe pear, thinly sliced
- 1/2 cup blue cheese, crumbled
- 2 tablespoons olive oil
- 1/4 cup pecans, toasted and chopped
- 1 tablespoon balsamic vinegar
- Salt and pepper to taste

INSTRUCTIONS:

1. In a large salad bowl, combine the arugula, thinly sliced pear, crumbled blue cheese, and toasted pecans.
2. In a small bowl, whisk together olive oil and balsamic vinegar. Season with salt and pepper.
3. Drizzle the dressing over the salad and toss gently to coat the ingredients evenly.
4. Serve immediately, offering a harmonious blend of peppery arugula, sweet pear, creamy blue cheese, and crunchy pecans.

NUTRITIONAL INFORMATION (PER SERVING):

Calories: 220 | Carbs: 10g | Fiber: 3g | Net Carbs: 7g
Protein: 6g | Fats: 18g

Mediterranean Chef Salad

Prep Time: 15 Minutes | **Cook Time:** 0 Minutes | **Serves:** 4

INGREDIENTS:

- 6 cups mixed greens (lettuce, spinach, arugula)
- 1 cup cherry tomatoes, halved
- 1 cucumber, sliced
- 1/2 red onion, thinly sliced
- 1/2 cup Kalamata olives, pitted
- 1/2 cup feta cheese, crumbled
- 1/4 cup extra virgin olive oil
- 2 tablespoons red wine vinegar
- 1 teaspoon dried oregano
- Salt and pepper to taste
- 4 hard-boiled eggs, quartered
- 8 slices of deli turkey or chicken, rolled and sliced

INSTRUCTIONS:

1. In a large salad bowl, combine mixed greens, cherry tomatoes, cucumber slices, red onion, Kalamata olives, and crumbled feta cheese.

2. In a small bowl, whisk together extra virgin olive oil, red wine vinegar, dried oregano, salt, and pepper to make the dressing.
3. Drizzle the dressing over the salad and toss to combine.
4. Arrange the quartered hard-boiled eggs and rolled deli turkey or chicken slices on top of the salad.
5. Serve immediately, offering a flavorful and refreshing Mediterranean twist to the traditional chef salad.

Calories: 320 | Carbs: 8g | Fiber: 3g | Net Carbs: 5g
Protein: 20g | Fats: 24g

Roasted Beet and Walnut Salad

Prep Time: 10 Minutes | **Cook Time:** 45 Minutes | **Serves:** 4

INGREDIENTS:

- 4 medium beets, roasted, peeled, and diced
- 4 cups mixed salad greens
- 1/2 cup walnuts, toasted and chopped
- 1/4 cup goat cheese, crumbled
- 2 tablespoons balsamic vinegar
- 2 tablespoons extra virgin olive oil
- Salt and pepper to taste

INSTRUCTIONS:

1. If not using pre-cooked beets, wrap whole beets in foil and roast in a preheated 400°F (200°C) oven for about 45 minutes, or until tender. Once cooled, peel and dice the beets.
2. In a large salad bowl, combine the mixed salad greens, diced roasted beets, toasted walnuts, and crumbled goat cheese.
3. In a small bowl, whisk together balsamic vinegar, extra virgin olive oil, salt, and pepper to create the dressing.
4. Drizzle the dressing over the salad and toss gently to combine.
5. Serve immediately, enjoying the earthy flavors of the beets with the creamy goat cheese and crunchy walnuts.

Calories: 260 | Carbs: 12g | Fiber: 3g | Net Carbs: 9g
Protein: 8g | Fats: 22g

Five-Layer Salad

Prep Time: 20 Minutes | **Cook Time:** 0 Minute | **Serves:** 6

INGREDIENTS:

- 4 cups chopped romaine lettuce
- 2 cups diced tomatoes
- 2 cups diced cucumbers
- 1 cup shredded cheddar cheese
- 1 cup cooked bacon, crumbled
- 1 cup mayonnaise, low-carb
- 1 tablespoon apple cider vinegar
- 1 teaspoon erythritol or other low-carb sweetener
- Salt and pepper to taste

INSTRUCTIONS:

1. In a large glass bowl or trifle dish, create the first layer with chopped romaine lettuce.
2. Add a layer of diced tomatoes, followed by a layer of diced cucumbers.
3. Sprinkle shredded cheddar cheese as the next layer, then top with crumbled cooked bacon.
4. In a small bowl, mix mayonnaise, apple cider vinegar, erythritol, salt, and pepper to make the dressing.
5. Spread the dressing evenly over the top layer, covering the salad completely.
6. Cover and chill in the refrigerator for at least an hour before serving to allow the flavors to meld.
7. Serve chilled, scooping down through the layers to get a bit of each in every serving.

Calories: 400 | Carbs: 6g | Fiber: 2g | Net Carbs: 4g
Protein: 12g | Fats: 36g

Asparagus and Parmesan Salad

Prep Time: 10 Minutes | **Cook Time:** 5 Minutes | **Serves:** 4

- ❖ 1 lb fresh asparagus, trimmed
- ❖ 1/4 cup shaved Parmesan cheese
- ❖ 2 tablespoons extra virgin olive oil
- ❖ 1 tablespoon lemon juice
- ❖ Salt and pepper to taste
- ❖ Lemon zest for garnish

INSTRUCTIONS:

1. Blanch the asparagus in boiling water for 2-3 minutes until bright green and slightly tender. Immediately transfer to an ice bath to stop the cooking process.
2. Once cooled, drain and arrange the asparagus on a serving platter.
3. Drizzle extra virgin olive oil and lemon juice over the asparagus. Season with salt and pepper.
4. Sprinkle shaved Parmesan cheese evenly over the asparagus.
5. Garnish with lemon zest before serving.

NUTRITIONAL INFORMATION (PER SERVING):

Calories: 120 | Carbs: 4g | Fiber: 2g | Net Carbs: 2g Protein: 5g | Fats: 10g

Tomato, Mozzarella, and Basil Salad

Prep Time: 10 Minutes | **Cook Time:** 0 Minute | **Serves:** 4

INGREDIENTS:

- ❖ 4 large ripe tomatoes, sliced
- ❖ 8 oz fresh mozzarella cheese, sliced
- ❖ 1/4 cup fresh basil leaves
- ❖ 2 tablespoons extra virgin olive oil
- ❖ 1 tablespoon balsamic vinegar (optional)
- ❖ Salt and pepper to taste

INSTRUCTIONS:

1. Arrange the tomato and mozzarella slices alternately on a platter, slightly overlapping each other.
2. Tuck fresh basil leaves between the tomato and mozzarella slices.
3. Drizzle extra virgin olive oil (and balsamic vinegar if using) over the arranged slices.
4. Season with salt and pepper to taste.

5. Serve immediately, enjoying the fresh and classic flavors of this simple salad.

NUTRITIONAL INFORMATION (PER SERVING):

Calories: 250 | Carbs: 6g | Fiber: 1g | Net Carbs: 5g Protein: 15g | Fats: 20g

Zucchini Noodle Caprese Salad

Prep Time: 15 Minutes | **Cook Time:** 0 Minute | **Serves:** 4

INGREDIENTS:

- ❖ 2 large zucchinis, spiralized into noodles
- ❖ 1 cup cherry tomatoes, halved
- ❖ 8 oz fresh mozzarella balls (bocconcini), halved
- ❖ 1/4 cup fresh basil leaves, chopped
- ❖ 2 tablespoons extra virgin olive oil
- ❖ 1 tablespoon white balsamic vinegar or regular balsamic vinegar
- ❖ Salt and pepper to taste

INSTRUCTIONS:

1. Place the spiralized zucchini noodles in a large salad bowl.
2. Add the halved cherry tomatoes, mozzarella balls, and chopped basil to the bowl with the zucchini noodles.
3. In a small bowl, whisk together extra virgin olive oil and balsamic vinegar. Season with salt and pepper.
4. Pour the dressing over the salad ingredients and gently toss to combine, ensuring the zucchini noodles and other components are well-coated with the dressing.
5. Serve immediately, offering a light and refreshing take on the traditional Caprese salad, perfect for a low-carb diet.

NUTRITIONAL INFORMATION (PER SERVING):

Calories: 220 | Carbs: 6g | Fiber: 2g | Net Carbs: 4g Protein: 12g | Fats: 16g

- 2 cups cooked chicken, shredded
- 1 cup carrots, grated
- 1/2 cup cashews, roasted and chopped
- 1/4 cup green onions, chopped
- 1/4 cup cilantro, chopped
- 2 tablespoons sesame oil
- 1 tablespoon soy sauce or tamari
- 1 tablespoon rice vinegar
- 1 teaspoon ginger, grated
- Salt and pepper to taste

Grilled Vegetable Salad with Herb Dressing

Prep Time: 15 Minutes | **Cook Time:** 10 Minutes | **Serves:** 4

INGREDIENTS:

Ingredients for Salad:

- 1 zucchini, sliced lengthwise
- 1 yellow squash, sliced lengthwise
- 1 red bell pepper, quartered
- 1 yellow bell pepper, quartered
- 1 eggplant, sliced into rounds
- 2 tablespoons olive oil
- Salt and pepper to taste

Ingredients for Herb Dressing:

- 1/4 cup olive oil
- 2 tablespoons lemon juice
- 1 tablespoon fresh parsley, finely chopped
- 1 tablespoon fresh basil, finely chopped
- 1 clove garlic, minced
- Salt and pepper to taste

INGREDIENTS: (Carrot and Cashew Chicken Salad)

INSTRUCTIONS:

1. Preheat a grill to medium-high heat. Brush the sliced vegetables with olive oil and season with salt and pepper.
2. Grill the vegetables for 3-4 minutes on each side until they are tender and have grill marks.
3. In a small bowl, whisk together the ingredients for the herb dressing until well combined.
4. Arrange the grilled vegetables on a serving platter and drizzle with the herb dressing.
5. Serve the salad warm or at room temperature.

NUTRITIONAL INFORMATION (PER SERVING):

Calories: 200 | Carbs: 12g | Fiber: 5g | Net Carbs: 7g

Protein: 3g | Fats: 16g

INSTRUCTIONS: (Carrot and Cashew Chicken Salad)

1. In a large bowl, combine the shredded chicken, grated carrots, roasted cashews, green onions, and cilantro.
2. In a small bowl, whisk together sesame oil, soy sauce, rice vinegar, and grated ginger to create the dressing.
3. Pour the dressing over the chicken mixture and toss to combine.
4. Season with salt and pepper to taste.
5. Serve the salad chilled or at room temperature.

NUTRITIONAL INFORMATION (PER SERVING):

Calories: 280 | Carbs: 10g | Fiber: 2g | Net Carbs: 8g

Protein: 25g | Fats: 6g

Carrot and Cashew Chicken Salad

Prep Time: 20 Minutes | **Cook Time:** 0 Minute | **Serves:** 4

Chicken, Avocado, and Spinach Salad

Prep Time: 15 Minutes | **Cook Time:** 0 Minutes | **Serves:** 4

INGREDIENTS:

- 2 cups cooked chicken, diced
- 2 avocados, diced
- 4 cups baby spinach
- 1/2 red onion, thinly sliced
- 1/4 cup almonds, slivered
- 2 tablespoons olive oil
- 1 tablespoon balsamic vinegar
- Salt and pepper to taste

INSTRUCTIONS:

1. In a large salad bowl, combine baby spinach, diced chicken, diced avocados, thinly sliced red onion, and slivered almonds.
2. In a small bowl, whisk together olive oil and balsamic

vinegar to create the dressing.

3. Drizzle the dressing over the salad and toss gently to combine.
4. Season with salt and pepper to taste.
5. Serve immediately, offering a hearty and nutritious salad perfect for a meal.

Calories: 350 | Carbs: 12g | Fiber: 7g | Net Carbs: 5g

Protein: 25g | Fats: 24g

BLT Cauliflower Salad

Prep Time: 15 Minutes | **Cook Time:** 10 Minutes | **Serves:** 4

INGREDIENTS:

- 1 large head of cauliflower, cut into bite-sized florets
- 6 slices of bacon, cooked and crumbled
- 1 cup cherry tomatoes, halved
- 1/4 cup mayonnaise, low-carb
- 2 cups mixed salad greens or chopped lettuce
- 2 tablespoons apple cider vinegar
- 1 teaspoon Dijon mustard
- Salt and pepper to taste

INSTRUCTIONS:

1. Steam the cauliflower florets until tender but still crisp, about 5-7 minutes. Allow to cool.
2. In a large mixing bowl, combine the cooled cauliflower, crumbled bacon, cherry tomatoes, and salad greens.
3. In a small bowl, whisk together mayonnaise, apple cider vinegar, Dijon mustard, salt, and pepper to create the dressing.
4. Pour the dressing over the salad ingredients and toss gently to coat.
5. Chill in the refrigerator for at least 30 minutes before serving to allow flavors to meld.

NUTRITIONAL INFORMATION (PER SERVING):

Calories: 220 | Carbs: 8g | Fiber: 3g | Net Carbs: 5g

Protein: 8g | Fats: 18g

Spicy Thai Beef Salad

Prep Time: 20 Minutes | **Cook Time:** 10 Minutes | **Serves:** 4

INGREDIENTS:

- 1 lb beef sirloin, thinly sliced
- 4 cups mixed salad greens
- 1 cucumber, sliced
- 1/2 red onion, thinly sliced
- 1/4 cup fresh cilantro, chopped
- 1/4 cup fresh mint, chopped

For the Dressing/Marinade:

- 2 tablespoons fish sauce
- 2 tablespoons lime juice
- 1 tablespoon soy sauce or tamari
- 1 tablespoon erythritol or other low-carb sweetener
- 1 teaspoon chili flakes (adjust to taste)
- 2 cloves garlic, minced

INSTRUCTIONS:

1. Combine all the dressing ingredients in a bowl. Reserve half for the salad and use the other half to marinate the beef for at least 30 minutes.
2. Grill or pan-fry the beef over high heat until cooked to your preference. Allow to rest, then slice thinly.
3. In a large salad bowl, combine the salad greens, cucumber, red onion, cilantro, and mint.
4. Add the cooked beef to the salad.
5. Drizzle the reserved dressing over the salad and toss gently to combine.
6. Serve immediately, garnished with additional herbs if desired.

NUTRITIONAL INFORMATION (PER SERVING):

Calories: 250 | Carbs: 6g | Fiber: 1g | Net Carbs: 5g

Protein: 25g | Fats: 14g

Roasted Cauliflower and Chickpea Salad

Prep Time: 15 Minutes | **Cook Time:** 20 Minutes | **Serves:** 4

INGREDIENTS:

- 1 large head of cauliflower, cut into florets
- 2 tablespoons olive oil
- 1 teaspoon ground cumin

- ❖ 1 can (14 oz) chickpeas, drained and rinsed (use sparingly for a lower carb option)
- ❖ 1/4 cup tahini
- ❖ Salt and pepper to taste
- ❖ 4 cups mixed salad greens
- ❖ 2 tablespoons lemon juice

INSTRUCTIONS:

1. Preheat your oven to 425°F (220°C). Toss cauliflower florets and chickpeas with olive oil, cumin, salt, and pepper. Spread on a baking sheet and roast for 20 minutes, until the cauliflower is tender and golden.
2. In a large salad bowl, combine the roasted cauliflower and chickpeas with the mixed salad greens.
3. In a small bowl, whisk together tahini, lemon juice, minced garlic, and water (as needed) to create a dressing. Season with salt and pepper.
4. Drizzle the dressing over the salad and toss gently to combine, ensuring all the ingredients are well coated.
5. Serve the salad immediately, or allow it to chill in the refrigerator for a short time to let the flavors meld together.

NUTRITIONAL INFORMATION (PER SERVING):

Calories: 260 | Carbs: 18g | Fiber: 6g | Net Carbs: 12g
Protein: 9g | Fats: 18g

Sweet Beet Grain Bowl

Prep Time: 20 Minutes | **Cook Time:** 40 Minutes | **Serves:** 4

INGREDIENTS:

- ❖ 4 medium beets, roasted and diced
- ❖ 2 cups cauliflower rice, cooked
- ❖ 1 cup arugula
- ❖ 1/2 cup walnuts, chopped
- ❖ 1/2 cup feta cheese, crumbled
- ❖ 2 tablespoons olive oil
- ❖ 1 tablespoon balsamic vinegar
- ❖ Salt and pepper to taste

INSTRUCTIONS:

1. Preheat your oven to 400°F (200°C). Wrap beets in foil and roast until tender, about 40 minutes. Let cool, peel, and dice.
2. Prepare the cauliflower rice according to package instructions or by sautéing in a pan until tender.
3. In a large bowl, combine the roasted beets, cooked cauliflower rice, arugula, walnuts, and feta cheese.
4. In a small bowl, whisk together olive oil, balsamic vinegar, salt, and pepper to make the dressing.
5. Drizzle the dressing over the salad and toss gently to combine.

NUTRITIONAL INFORMATION (PER SERVING):

Calories: 250 | Carbs: 15g | Fiber: 5g | Net Carbs: 10g
Protein: 8g | Fats: 18g

Raw Corn Salad with Black-Eyed Peas

Prep Time: 15 Minutes | **Cook Time:** 0 Minute | **Serves:** 6

INGREDIENTS:

- ❖ 2 cups fresh corn kernels (or substitute with chopped bell peppers for a lower carb option)
- ❖ 1 can black-eyed peas, rinsed and drained
- ❖ 1 cup cherry tomatoes, halved
- ❖ 1 avocado, diced
- ❖ 1/4 cup red onion, finely chopped
- ❖ 2 tablespoons cilantro, chopped
- ❖ Juice of 1 lime
- ❖ 2 tablespoons olive oil
- ❖ Salt and pepper to taste

INSTRUCTIONS:

1. In a large bowl, combine corn kernels (or bell pepper), black-eyed peas, cherry tomatoes, avocado, and red onion.
2. Add chopped cilantro to the bowl.
3. In a small bowl, whisk together lime juice, olive oil, salt, and pepper to create the dressing.
4. Pour the dressing over the salad and toss gently to coat evenly.
5. Serve immediately or chill in the refrigerator to enhance the flavors.

NUTRITIONAL INFORMATION (PER SERVING):

Calories: 180 | Carbs: 22g | Fiber: 6g | Net Carbs: 16g
Protein: 6g | Fats: 8g

Greek Salad with Marinated Feta

Prep Time: 15 Minutes | **Cook Time:** 0 Minutes | **Serves:** 4

INGREDIENTS:

- ❖ 2 cups cucumber, diced
- ❖ 2 cups cherry tomatoes, halved
- ❖ 1/2 cup Kalamata olives
- ❖ 1/4 cup red onion, thinly sliced
- ❖ 1 cup feta cheese, cubed
- ❖ 1/4 cup olive oil (for marinating feta)
- ❖ 1 tablespoon lemon juice
- ❖ 1 teaspoon dried oregano
- ❖ 2 tablespoons olive oil (for salad)
- ❖ 1 tablespoon red wine vinegar
- ❖ Salt and pepper to taste

INSTRUCTIONS:

1. Marinate cubed feta cheese in 1/4 cup olive oil, lemon juice, and dried oregano for at least 1 hour.
2. In a large salad bowl, combine cucumber, cherry tomatoes, Kalamata olives, and red onion.
3. Add the marinated feta cheese to the salad.
4. In a small bowl, whisk together 2 tablespoons olive oil, red wine vinegar, salt, and pepper to make the dressing.
5. Pour the dressing over the salad and toss gently to combine.

NUTRITIONAL INFORMATION (PER SERVING):

Calories: 250 | Carbs: 10g | Fiber: 2g | Net Carbs: 8g
Protein: 7g | Fats: 21g

Watermelon and Feta Salad with Mint

Prep Time: 15 Minutes | **Cook Time:** 0 Minutes | **Serves:** 4

INGREDIENTS:

- ❖ 4 cups cubed watermelon
- ❖ 1/2 cup crumbled feta cheese
- ❖ 2 tablespoons chopped fresh mint leaves
- ❖ Salt and pepper to taste
- ❖ 1 tablespoon extra virgin olive oil

INSTRUCTIONS:

1. In a large bowl, combine the cubed watermelon, crumbled feta cheese, and chopped fresh mint leaves.
2. Drizzle the extra virgin olive oil over the salad and toss gently to coat.
3. Season with salt and pepper to taste.
4. Serve immediately or chill in the refrigerator until ready to serve.

NUTRITIONAL INFORMATION (PER SERVING):

Calories: 120 | Carbs: 10g | Fiber: 1g | Net Carbs: 9g
Protein: 4g | Fats: 7g

Brussels Sprout and Pecan Salad

Prep Time: 20 Minutes | **Cook Time:** 5 Minutes | **Serves:** 4

INGREDIENTS:

- ❖ 1 lb Brussels sprouts, trimmed and thinly sliced
- ❖ 1/2 cup chopped pecans, toasted
- ❖ 1/4 cup grated Parmesan cheese
- ❖ 1 tablespoon apple cider vinegar
- ❖ 1 teaspoon Dijon mustard
- ❖ Salt and pepper to taste
- ❖ 2 tablespoons extra virgin olive oil

INSTRUCTIONS:

1. In a large bowl, combine the thinly sliced Brussels sprouts, chopped toasted pecans, and grated Parmesan cheese.
2. In a small bowl, whisk together the extra virgin olive oil, apple cider vinegar, Dijon mustard, salt, and pepper to make the dressing.
3. Pour the dressing over the salad and toss until well coated.
4. Serve immediately or refrigerate until ready to serve.

NUTRITIONAL INFORMATION (PER SERVING):

Calories: 220 | Carbs: 9g | Fiber: 4g | Net Carbs: 5g
Protein: 6g | Fats: 18g

Endive and Apple Salad with Walnuts

Prep Time: 15 Minutes | **Cook Time:** 0 Minute | **Serves:** 4

INGREDIENTS:

- ❖ 2 large endives, leaves separated
- ❖ 2 Granny Smith apples, thinly sliced
- ❖ 1/2 cup chopped walnuts, toasted
- ❖ 1/4 cup crumbled blue cheese (optional)
- ❖ 2 tablespoons extra virgin olive oil
- ❖ 1 tablespoon balsamic vinegar
- ❖ 1 teaspoon honey (optional)
- ❖ Salt and pepper to taste

INSTRUCTIONS:

1. Arrange the endive leaves on a serving platter.
2. Top with thinly sliced Granny Smith apples and chopped toasted walnuts.
3. If using, sprinkle crumbled blue cheese over the salad.
4. In a small bowl, whisk together the extra virgin olive oil, balsamic vinegar, honey (if using), salt, and pepper to make the dressing.
5. Drizzle the dressing over the salad just before serving.

NUTRITIONAL INFORMATION (PER SERVING):

Calories: 200 | Carbs: 15g | Fiber: 5g | Net Carbs: 10g
Protein: 4g | Fats: 15g

Radish and Cucumber Salad with Lemon Vinaigrette

Prep Time: 10 Minutes | **Cook Time:** 0 Minute | **Serves:** 4

INGREDIENTS:

- ❖ 1 bunch radishes, thinly sliced
- ❖ 1 English cucumber, thinly sliced
- ❖ 2 tablespoons chopped fresh dill
- ❖ 2 tablespoons extra virgin olive oil
- ❖ 1 tablespoon freshly squeezed lemon juice
- ❖ Salt and pepper to taste

INSTRUCTIONS:

1. In a large bowl, combine the thinly sliced radishes and cucumber.
2. In a small bowl, whisk together the chopped fresh dill, extra virgin olive oil, lemon juice, salt, and pepper to make the vinaigrette.
3. Pour the vinaigrette over the salad and toss until well coated.
4. Serve immediately or refrigerate until ready to serve.

NUTRITIONAL INFORMATION (PER SERVING):

Calories: 70 | Carbs: 4g | Fiber: 1g | Net Carbs: 3g
Protein: 1g | Fats: 6g

Chapter 12
Snacks and Appetizers

Avocado and Salsa Stuffed Mini Peppers

Prep Time: 10 Minutes | **Cook Time:** 20 Minutes |
Serves: 4

INGREDIENTS:

- 12 mini bell peppers, halved and seeded
- 1 cup cream cheese, softened
- 1/4 cup salsa of choice
- 1 ripe avocado, diced
- 2 tablespoons chopped cilantro (optional)
- Everything bagel seasoning (for garnish)

INSTRUCTIONS:

1. In a bowl, mix the cream cheese and salsa until well combined. Fold in the diced avocado and cilantro if using.
2. Stuff each mini pepper half with the cream cheese mixture.
3. Sprinkle everything bagel seasoning over the stuffed peppers for added flavor.
4. For a warm version, bake the stuffed peppers on a baking sheet in a preheated oven at 350°F for 15-20 minutes or until the peppers are tender.

NUTRITIONAL INFORMATION (PER SERVING):

Calories: 190 | Carbs: 6g | Fiber: 3g | Net Carbs: 5g
Protein: 4g | Fats: 17g

Zucchini Chips with Herbed Yogurt Dip

Prep Time: 10 Minutes | **Cook Time:** 30 Minutes |
Serves: 4

INGREDIENTS:

- 2 large zucchinis, thinly sliced
- 1 tablespoon olive oil
- Salt to taste
- 1 cup Greek yogurt
- 1 tablespoon fresh dill, chopped
- 1 tablespoon fresh chives, chopped
- 1 clove garlic, minced
- Juice of 1/2 lemon

INSTRUCTIONS:

1. Preheat your oven to 225°F. Line a baking sheet with parchment paper.
2. Toss zucchini slices with olive oil and salt. Arrange in a single layer on the baking sheet.
3. Bake for 20-30 minutes or until crispy and golden.
4. For the dip, combine Greek yogurt, dill, chives, garlic, and lemon juice in a bowl. Mix well.
5. Serve crispy zucchini chips with herbed yogurt dip.

NUTRITIONAL INFORMATION (PER SERVING):

Calories: 120 | Carbs: 10g | Fiber: 2g | Net Carbs: 8g
Protein: 6g | Fats: 7g

Eggplant Rollatini with Ricotta and Spinach

Prep Time: 20 Minutes | **Cook Time:** 40 Minutes |
Serves: 4

INGREDIENTS:

- 2 medium eggplants, sliced lengthwise (about 8 slices total)
- 1 cup ricotta cheese
- 1 cup spinach, chopped
- 1/2 cup grated Parmesan cheese
- 1 egg
- 2 cups marinara sauce
- 1/2 cup shredded mozzarella cheese
- Salt and pepper to taste
- 1 tablespoon olive oil

INSTRUCTIONS:

1. Start by preheating your oven to 375°F. Brush eggplant slices with olive oil, season with salt and pepper, and bake on a baking sheet for 15 minutes.
2. Mix ricotta, spinach, Parmesan, and egg in a bowl. Season with salt and pepper.
3. Spread a spoonful of ricotta mixture on each eggplant slice, roll up, and place seam-side down in a baking dish.
4. Cover with marinara sauce and sprinkle mozzarella on top.
5. Bake for 25 minutes or until cheese is bubbly and golden.

NUTRITIONAL INFORMATION (PER SERVING):

Calories: 320 | Carbs: 20g | Fiber: 6g | Net Carbs: 14g
Protein: 18g | Fats: 20g

Cauliflower Buffalo Bites

Prep Time: 15 Minutes | **Cook Time:** 35 Minutes | **Serves:** 4

INGREDIENTS:

- Fresh cauliflower cut into florets
- Almond flour for a low-carb option
- Eggs
- Spices including garlic powder, salt, and optional pepper
- Buffalo sauce, with a recommendation for Frank's Red Hot
- Avocado oil
- Green onions for garnish
- Your choice of dipping sauce

INSTRUCTIONS:

1. Start by preheating your oven and preparing a baking sheet with parchment paper.
2. Mix almond flour with spices in one bowl, and whisk eggs in another.
3. Dip cauliflower florets first in eggs, then coat with the almond flour mixture.
4. Arrange the florets on the baking sheet and bake until tender and slightly browned.
5. Combine avocado oil and buffalo sauce, then drizzle over the baked florets, garnishing with green onions before serving.

NUTRITIONAL INFORMATION (PER SERVING):

Calories: 150 | Carbs: 7g | Fiber: 3g | Net Carbs: 4g
Protein: 4g | Fats: 11g

Chicken Kabobs

Prep Time: 20 Minutes | **Cook Time:** 15 Minutes | **Serves:** 4

INGREDIENTS:

- 1 lb boneless, skinless chicken breasts, cut into chunks
- 1 bell pepper, cut into chunks
- 1 red onion, cut into chunks
- 8 cherry tomatoes
- 8 button mushrooms
- 2 tablespoons olive oil
- 2 tablespoons lemon juice
- 2 cloves garlic, minced
- 1 teaspoon dried oregano
- Salt and pepper to taste
- Wooden skewers, soaked in water for 30 minutes

INSTRUCTIONS:

1. In a large bowl, combine the olive oil, lemon juice, minced garlic, dried oregano, salt, and pepper.
2. Add the chicken chunks to the bowl and toss until evenly coated in the marinade. Allow the chicken to marinate for at least 15 minutes, or up to overnight in the refrigerator.
3. Preheat the grill or grill pan over medium-high heat.
4. Thread the marinated chicken, bell pepper, red onion, cherry tomatoes, and mushrooms onto the soaked wooden skewers, alternating the ingredients.
5. Grill the skewers for 10-15 minutes, turning occasionally, until the chicken is cooked through and the vegetables are tender.
6. Serve hot with your choice of side dishes or dipping sauces.

NUTRITIONAL INFORMATION (PER SERVING):

Calories: 250 | Carbs: 7g | Fiber: 2g | Net Carbs: 5g
Protein: 25g | Fats: 14g

Stuffed Mushrooms with Pesto and Feta

Prep Time: 15 Minutes | **Cook Time:** 20 Minutes | **Serves:** 4

INGREDIENTS:

- 16 large button mushrooms, stems removed and reserved
- 2 tablespoons olive oil
- 1/4 cup crumbled feta cheese
- 2 cloves garlic, minced
- 1/4 cup pesto sauce
- Salt and pepper to taste
- Fresh parsley for garnish (optional)

INSTRUCTIONS:

1. Preheat your oven to 375°F (190°C). Line a baking sheet with parchment paper.
2. Finely chop the reserved mushroom stems.
3. In a skillet, heat the olive oil over medium heat. Add

the minced garlic and chopped mushroom stems, and sauté until softened, about 3-4 minutes.

4. Remove the skillet from the heat and stir in the pesto sauce and crumbled feta cheese until well combined. Season with salt and pepper to taste.
5. Stuff each mushroom cap with the pesto-feta mixture and place them on the prepared baking sheet.
6. Bake in the preheated oven for 15-20 minutes, or until the mushrooms are tender and the filling is heated through.
7. Garnish with fresh parsley before serving, if desired.

NUTRITIONAL INFORMATION (PER SERVING):

Calories: 120 | Carbs: 4g | Fiber: 1g | Net Carbs: 3g
Protein: 3g | Fats: 10g

Cucumber and Smoked Salmon Canapés

Prep Time: 15 Minutes | **Cook Time:** 0 Minutes |
Serves: 4

INGREDIENTS:

- 1 English cucumber
- 4 oz smoked salmon, thinly sliced
- 1/4 cup cream cheese, softened
- 1 tablespoon fresh dill, chopped
- 1 tablespoon capers, drained
- Lemon zest, for garnish (optional)

INSTRUCTIONS:

1. Slice the cucumber into rounds, about 1/4 inch thick.
2. In a small bowl, mix together the softened cream cheese and chopped fresh dill.
3. Spread a thin layer of the cream cheese mixture onto each cucumber round.
4. Top each cucumber round with a slice of smoked salmon.
5. Garnish with capers and lemon zest, if desired.
6. Serve immediately or refrigerate until ready to serve.

NUTRITIONAL INFORMATION (PER SERVING):

Calories: 90 | Carbs: 2g | Fiber: 0g | Net Carbs: 2g
Protein: 6g | Fats: 6g

Prosciutto-Wrapped Asparagus Spears

Prep Time: 10 Minutes | **Cook Time:** 10 Minutes |
Serves: 4

INGREDIENTS:

- 1 lb asparagus spears, woody ends trimmed
- 4 oz thinly sliced prosciutto
- 1 tablespoon olive oil
- Salt and pepper to taste
- Balsamic glaze, for drizzling (optional)

INSTRUCTIONS:

1. Preheat your oven to 400°F (200°C). Line a baking sheet with parchment paper.
2. Toss the trimmed asparagus spears with olive oil, salt, and pepper.
3. Wrap each asparagus spear with a slice of prosciutto.
4. Place the wrapped asparagus spears on the prepared baking sheet.
5. Bake in the preheated oven for 8-10 minutes, or until the asparagus is tender and the prosciutto is crispy.
6. Drizzle with balsamic glaze before serving, if desired.

NUTRITIONAL INFORMATION (PER SERVING):

Calories: 100 | Carbs: 3g | Fiber: 1g | Net Carbs: 2g
Protein: 7g | Fats: 6g

Mini Bell Pepper Nachos

Prep Time: 15 Minutes | **Cook Time:** 10 Minutes |
Serves: 4

INGREDIENTS:

- 8 mini bell peppers, halved and seeded
- 1 cup shredded cheddar cheese
- 1/4 cup diced tomatoes
- 1/4 cup diced red onion
- 2 tablespoons sliced black olives
- 2 tablespoons chopped fresh cilantro
- 1 teaspoon taco seasoning
- Sour cream, for serving (optional)
- Guacamole, for serving (optional)

INSTRUCTIONS:

1. Preheat your oven to 400°F (200°C). Line a baking sheet with parchment paper.
2. Arrange the halved and seeded mini bell peppers on the prepared baking sheet.
3. Fill each pepper half with shredded cheddar cheese.
4. Top with diced tomatoes, diced red onion, sliced black olives, and chopped fresh cilantro.
5. Sprinkle taco seasoning over the top of each filled pepper half.
6. Bake in the preheated oven for 8-10 minutes, or until the cheese is melted and bubbly.
7. Serve hot with sour cream and guacamole, if desired.

NUTRITIONAL INFORMATION (PER SERVING):

Calories: 120 | Carbs: 5g | Fiber: 1g | Net Carbs: 4g
Protein: 6g | Fats: 8g

Baked Parmesan Crisps

Prep Time: 5 Minutes | **Cook Time:** 7 Minutes |
Serves: 4

INGREDIENTS:

- 1 cup grated Parmesan cheese
- 2 teaspoons almond flour

INSTRUCTIONS:

1. Start by preheating your oven to 375°F (190°C). Prepare two baking sheets by lining them with parchment paper or silicone mats to prevent sticking.
2. In a mixing bowl, combine the shredded Parmesan cheese with the almond flour. This helps to bind the cheese and create a more consistent crisp.
3. Place tablespoon-sized mounds of grated Parmesan cheese onto the prepared baking sheet, spacing them apart.
4. Flatten each mound slightly with the back of a spoon.
5. Bake in the preheated oven for 5-7 minutes, or until the crisps are golden brown and crispy.
6. Allow the crisps to cool on the baking sheet for a few minutes before transferring them to a wire rack to cool completely.

NUTRITIONAL INFORMATION (PER SERVING):

Calories: 80 | Carbs: 1g | Fiber: 0g | Net Carbs: 1g
Protein: 8g | Fats: 5g

Spiced Nuts Mix

Prep Time: 5 Minutes | **Cook Time:** 10 Minutes |
Serves: 4

INGREDIENTS:

- 1 cup mixed nuts (such as almonds, walnuts, pecans)
- 1 tablespoon melted butter or olive oil
- 1 teaspoon ground cumin
- 1/2 teaspoon chili powder
- 1/4 teaspoon garlic powder
- 1/4 teaspoon onion powder
- Salt to taste

INSTRUCTIONS:

1. Preheat your oven to 350°F (175°C). Line a baking sheet with parchment paper.
2. In a large bowl, toss together the mixed nuts, melted butter or olive oil, ground cumin, chili powder, garlic powder, onion powder, and salt until the nuts are evenly coated.
3. Spread the seasoned nuts in a single layer on the prepared baking sheet.
4. Bake in the preheated oven for 8-10 minutes, or until the nuts are lightly toasted and fragrant.
5. Allow the nuts to cool completely before serving or storing in an airtight container.

NUTRITIONAL INFORMATION (PER SERVING):

Calories: 220 | Carbs: 4g | Fiber: 2g | Net Carbs: 2g
Protein: 5g | Fats: 18g

Cheese Crisps with Avocado Dip

Prep Time: 10 Minutes | **Cook Time:** 10 Minutes |
Serves: 4

INGREDIENTS:

- 1 cup shredded cheddar cheese
- 1 cup shredded mozzarella cheese
- 1 avocado, pitted and peeled
- 1 tablespoon lime juice
- 1 tablespoon chopped fresh cilantro
- Salt and pepper to taste

INSTRUCTIONS:

1. Preheat your oven to 375°F (190°C). Line a baking sheet with parchment paper.
2. In a medium bowl, mix together the shredded cheddar cheese and shredded mozzarella cheese.
3. Spoon tablespoon-sized mounds of the cheese mixture onto the prepared baking sheet, spacing them apart.
4. Flatten each mound slightly with the back of a spoon to form rounds.
5. Bake in the preheated oven for 5-7 minutes, or until the crisps are golden brown and crispy.
6. Meanwhile, in a small bowl, mash the avocado with lime juice, chopped fresh cilantro, salt, and pepper to make the avocado dip.
7. Serve the cheese crisps warm with the avocado dip.

NUTRITIONAL INFORMATION (PER SERVING):

Calories: 220 | Carbs: 5g | Fiber: 3g | Net Carbs: 2g
Protein: 12g | Fats: 18g

Jalapeño Poppers Filled with Cream Cheese

Prep Time: 15 Minutes | **Cook Time:** 15 Minutes
Serves: 4

INGREDIENTS:

- 8 fresh jalapeño peppers
- 4 oz cream cheese, softened
- 1/4 cup shredded cheddar cheese
- 1/4 teaspoon garlic powder
- 1/4 teaspoon onion powder
- Salt and pepper to taste
- Bacon slices, halved (optional)

INSTRUCTIONS:

1. Preheat your oven to 375°F (190°C). Line a baking sheet with parchment paper.
2. Cut the jalapeño peppers in half lengthwise and remove the seeds and membranes.
3. In a small bowl, mix together the softened cream cheese, shredded cheddar cheese, garlic powder, onion powder, salt, and pepper.
4. Spoon the cream cheese mixture into the halved jalapeño peppers, filling each one.
5. If desired, wrap each stuffed jalapeño half with a half slice of bacon and secure with a toothpick.
6. Place the stuffed jalapeño halves on the prepared baking sheet.
7. Bake in the preheated oven for 12-15 minutes, or until the peppers are tender and the cheese is bubbly and lightly browned.
8. Serve hot as an appetizer or snack.

NUTRITIONAL INFORMATION (PER SERVING):

Calories: 110 | Carbs: 3g | Fiber: 1g | Net Carbs: 2g
Protein: 4g | Fats: 9g

Olive Tapenade on Cucumber Slices

Prep Time: 10 Minutes | **Cook Time:** 0 Minute
Serves: 4

INGREDIENTS:

- 1 cup pitted black olives
- 2 tablespoons capers
- 2 tablespoons chopped fresh parsley
- 1 tablespoon lemon juice
- 1 clove garlic, minced
- 2 tablespoons extra virgin olive oil
- Salt and pepper to taste
- 2 large cucumbers, sliced

INSTRUCTIONS:

1. In a food processor, combine the pitted black olives, capers, chopped fresh parsley, lemon juice, minced garlic, extra virgin olive oil, salt, and pepper.
2. Pulse until the mixture reaches your desired consistency, scraping down the sides as needed.
3. Arrange the cucumber slices on a serving platter.
4. Spoon a small amount of olive tapenade onto each cucumber slice.
5. Serve immediately as an appetizer or snack.

NUTRITIONAL INFORMATION (PER SERVING):

Calories: 90 | Carbs: 4g | Fiber: 2g | Net Carbs: 2g
Protein: 1g | Fats: 8g

Marinated Artichoke Hearts

Prep Time: 10 Minutes | **Cook Time:** 0 Minute
Serves: 4

- 1 can (14 oz) artichoke hearts, drained and quartered
- 2 tablespoons extra virgin olive oil
- 1 tablespoon balsamic vinegar
- 1 clove garlic, minced
- 1/2 teaspoon dried oregano
- Salt and pepper to taste
- Fresh parsley for garnish (optional)

INSTRUCTIONS:

1. In a medium bowl, whisk together the extra virgin olive oil, balsamic vinegar, minced garlic, dried oregano, salt, and pepper to make the marinade.
2. Add the drained and quartered artichoke hearts to the marinade and toss until evenly coated.
3. Cover the bowl and refrigerate for at least 1 hour to allow the flavors to meld.
4. Before serving, garnish with fresh parsley if desired.
5. Serve chilled as an appetizer or side dish.

NUTRITIONAL INFORMATION (PER SERVING):

Calories: 70 | Carbs: 3g | Fiber: 2g | Net Carbs: 1g
Protein: 1g | Fats: 6g

Ricotta and Herb Stuffed Cherry Tomatoes

Prep Time: 15 Minutes | **Cook Time:** 0 Minute | **Serves:** 4

INGREDIENTS:

- 1/2 cup ricotta cheese
- 1 tablespoon chopped fresh basil
- 1 teaspoon lemon zest
- 16 cherry tomatoes
- tablespoon chopped fresh parsley
- Salt and pepper to taste

INSTRUCTIONS:

1. Cut the tops off of the cherry tomatoes and scoop out the seeds and pulp.
2. In a small bowl, mix together the ricotta cheese, chopped fresh basil, chopped fresh parsley, lemon zest, salt, and pepper.
3. Spoon the ricotta mixture into the hollowed-out cherry tomatoes.
4. Serve immediately as an appetizer or snack.

NUTRITIONAL INFORMATION (PER SERVING):

Calories: 50 | Carbs: 3g | Fiber: 1g | Net Carbs: 2g
Protein: 3g | Fats: 3g

Peanut Butter Protein Bites

Prep Time: 15 Minutes | **Cook Time:** 0 Minute | **Serves:** 4

INGREDIENTS:

- 1/2 cup natural peanut butter
- 1/4 cup almond flour
- 2 tablespoons unsweetened cocoa powder
- 2 tablespoons low-carb sweetener (such as erythritol or stevia)
- 1 teaspoon vanilla extract
- Pinch of salt

INSTRUCTIONS:

1. In a mixing bowl, combine the natural peanut butter, almond flour, unsweetened cocoa powder, low-carb sweetener, vanilla extract, and a pinch of salt.
2. Mix until well combined and a dough forms.
3. Roll the dough into tablespoon-sized balls.
4. Refrigerate the peanut butter protein bites for at least 30 minutes before serving.

NUTRITIONAL INFORMATION (PER SERVING):

Calories: 170 | Carbs: 6g | Fiber: 2g | Net Carbs: 4g
Protein: 7g | Fats: 14g

Roasted Garlic and Chive Dip with Vegetable Sticks

Prep Time: 10 Minutes | **Cook Time:** 30 Minutes | **Serves:** 4

INGREDIENTS:

- 1 bulb garlic
- 2 teaspoons olive oil
- 1 cup sour cream
- 1/4 cup mayonnaise

* 2 tablespoons chopped fresh chives
* Salt and pepper to taste
* Assorted vegetable sticks (such as carrots, celery, bell peppers, cucumber) for serving

INSTRUCTIONS:

1. Start by preheating your oven to 400°F (200°C).
2. Slice the top off of the garlic bulb to expose the cloves.
3. Drizzle the exposed cloves with olive oil and wrap the bulb in aluminum foil.
4. Roast the garlic in the preheated oven for 25-30 minutes, or until the cloves are soft and golden brown.
5. Allow the roasted garlic to cool slightly, then squeeze the cloves out of the skins into a mixing bowl.
6. Add the sour cream, mayonnaise, chopped fresh chives, salt, and pepper to the bowl with the roasted garlic cloves.
7. Stir until well combined and creamy.
8. Serve the roasted garlic and chive dip with assorted vegetable sticks for dipping.

NUTRITIONAL INFORMATION (PER SERVING):

Calories: 180 | Carbs: 6g | Fiber: 1g | Net Carbs: 5g
Protein: 2g | Fats: 17g

Deviled Eggs with Smoked Paprika

Prep Time: 15 Minutes | **Cook Time:** 12 Minutes |
Serves: 4

INGREDIENTS:

* 4 large eggs
* 2 tablespoons mayonnaise
* 1 teaspoon Dijon mustard
* 1/2 teaspoon white vinegar
* Salt and pepper to taste
* Smoked paprika for garnish
* Fresh chives for garnish

INSTRUCTIONS:

1. Place the eggs in a single layer in a saucepan and cover with water.
2. Bring the water to a boil over medium-high heat.
3. Once boiling, remove the saucepan from the heat, cover, and let the eggs sit in the hot water for 10-12 minutes.
4. Drain the hot water and transfer the eggs to a bowl of ice water to cool.
5. Once cooled, peel the eggs and cut them in half lengthwise. Remove the yolks and place them in a separate bowl.
6. Mash the egg yolks with a fork and add the mayonnaise, Dijon mustard, white vinegar, salt, and pepper. Mix until smooth.
7. Spoon or pipe the yolk mixture back into the egg white halves.
8. Sprinkle the deviled eggs with smoked paprika and garnish with fresh chives before serving.

NUTRITIONAL INFORMATION (PER SERVING):

Calories: 110 | Carbs: 1g | Fiber: 0g | Net Carbs: 1g
Protein: 6g | Fats: 9g

Caprese Skewers with Balsamic Glaze

Prep Time: 15 Minutes | **Cook Time:** 0 Minute |
Serves: 4

INGREDIENTS:

* 12 cherry tomatoes
* 12 fresh mozzarella balls (bocconcini)
* 12 fresh basil leaves
* Balsamic glaze for drizzling

INSTRUCTIONS:

1. Thread a cherry tomato, a fresh mozzarella ball, and a fresh basil leaf onto each skewer.
2. Arrange the skewers on a serving platter.
3. Drizzle the skewers with balsamic glaze just before serving.

NUTRITIONAL INFORMATION (PER SERVING):

Calories: 120 | Carbs: 3g | Fiber: 0g | Net Carbs: 3g
Protein: 7g | Fats: 8g

Vegetable Kabobs with Mustard Dip

Prep Time: 20 Minutes | **Cook Time:** 10 Minutes |
Serves: 4

INGREDIENTS:

- 1 zucchini, sliced into rounds
- 1 yellow squash, sliced into rounds
- 1 bell pepper, cut into chunks
- 1 red onion, cut into chunks
- 8 cherry tomatoes
- 8 button mushrooms
- 2 tablespoons olive oil
- Salt and pepper to taste
- Wooden skewers, soaked in water for 30 minutes

For Mustard Dip:

- 1/4 cup mayonnaise
- 1 tablespoon Dijon mustard
- 1 tablespoon lemon juice
- 1 clove garlic, minced
- Salt and pepper to taste

INSTRUCTIONS:

1. Preheat a grill or grill pan over medium-high heat.
2. In a large bowl, toss together the sliced zucchini, yellow squash, bell pepper chunks, red onion chunks, cherry tomatoes, and button mushrooms with olive oil, salt, and pepper.
3. Thread the mixed vegetables onto the soaked wooden skewers, alternating the ingredients.
4. Grill the vegetable skewers for 8-10 minutes, turning occasionally, until the vegetables are tender and slightly charred.
5. Meanwhile, prepare the mustard dip by combining the mayonnaise, Dijon mustard, lemon juice, minced garlic, salt, and pepper in a small bowl.
6. Serve the grilled vegetable kabobs hot with the mustard dip on the side.

NUTRITIONAL INFORMATION (PER SERVING):

Calories: 180 | Carbs: 10g | Fiber: 3g | Net Carbs: 7g
Protein: 2g | Fats: 15g

Spinach and Feta Stuffed Portobello Caps

Prep Time: 15 Minutes | **Cook Time:** 20 Minutes |
Serves: 4

INGREDIENTS:

- 4 large portobello mushroom caps
- 2 cups fresh spinach, chopped
- 2 tablespoons olive oil
- 2 cloves garlic, minced
- 1/2 cup crumbled feta cheese
- Salt and pepper to taste
- Fresh parsley for garnish (optional)

INSTRUCTIONS:

1. Preheat your oven to 375°F (190°C). Line a baking sheet with parchment paper.
2. Clean the portobello mushroom caps and remove the stems.
3. In a skillet, heat olive oil over medium heat. Add the minced garlic and cook until fragrant, about 1 minute.
4. Add the chopped fresh spinach to the skillet and cook until wilted, about 2-3 minutes. Season with salt and pepper to taste.
5. Remove the skillet from the heat and stir in the crumbled feta cheese until well combined.
6. Spoon the spinach and feta mixture into the cavity of each portobello mushroom cap.
7. Place the stuffed mushroom caps on the prepared baking sheet.
8. Bake in the preheated oven for 15-20 minutes, or until the mushrooms are tender and the filling is heated through.
9. Garnish with fresh parsley before serving, if desired.

NUTRITIONAL INFORMATION (PER SERVING):

Calories: 140 | Carbs: 5g | Fiber: 2g | Net Carbs: 3g
Protein: 5g | Fats: 11g

Shrimp Cocktail with Sugar-Free Sauce

Prep Time: 10 Minutes | **Cook Time:** 5 Minutes |
Serves: 4

INGREDIENTS:

- 1 lb cooked shrimp, peeled and devcined
- 1/2 cup sugar-free ketchup
- 1 tablespoon prepared horseradish
- 1 tablespoon lemon juice
- 1 teaspoon Worcestershire sauce
- Dash of hot sauce (optional)
- Lemon wedges for garnish
- Fresh parsley for garnish (optional)

INSTRUCTIONS:

1. In a small bowl, mix together the sugar-free ketchup, prepared horseradish, lemon juice, Worcestershire sauce, and hot sauce (if using) to make the cocktail sauce.
2. Arrange the cooked shrimp on a serving platter.
3. Serve the shrimp cocktail with the sugar-free cocktail sauce on the side.
4. Garnish with lemon wedges and fresh parsley, if desired.

NUTRITIONAL INFORMATION (PER SERVING):

Calories: 150 | Carbs: 5g | Fiber: 0g | Net Carbs: 5g

Protein: 25g | Fats: 2g

Savory Pumpkin Seeds

Prep Time: 10 Minutes | **Cook Time:** 20 Minutes | **Serves:** 4

INGREDIENTS:

- 2 cups raw pumpkin seeds (pepitas), rinsed and dried
- 1 tablespoon olive oil
- 1 teaspoon garlic powder
- 1 teaspoon onion powder
- 1/2 teaspoon smoked paprika
- Salt to taste

INSTRUCTIONS:

1. Preheat your oven to 300°F (150°C). Line a baking sheet with parchment paper.
2. In a mixing bowl, toss together the raw pumpkin seeds, olive oil, garlic powder, onion powder, smoked paprika, and salt until the seeds are evenly coated.
3. Spread the seasoned pumpkin seeds in a single layer on the prepared baking sheet.
4. Bake in the preheated oven for 15-20 minutes, stirring occasionally, until the pumpkin seeds are golden brown and crispy.
5. Allow the pumpkin seeds to cool completely before serving or storing in an airtight container.

NUTRITIONAL INFORMATION (PER SERVING):

Calories: 180 | Carbs: 3g | Fiber: 1g | Net Carbs: 2g

Protein: 10g | Fats: 15g

Greek Salad Bites

Prep Time: 15 Minutes | **Cook Time:** 0 Minute | **Serves:** 4

INGREDIENTS:

- 1 cup cherry tomatoes, halved
- 1/2 cucumber, diced
- 1/2 cup Kalamata olives, pitted and halved
- 1/4 cup crumbled feta cheese
- 2 tablespoons extra virgin olive oil
- 1 tablespoon red wine vinegar
- 1 teaspoon dried oregano
- Salt and pepper to taste
- Fresh parsley for garnish (optional)

INSTRUCTIONS:

1. In a large bowl, combine the halved cherry tomatoes, diced cucumber, halved Kalamata olives, and crumbled feta cheese.
2. In a small bowl, whisk together the extra virgin olive oil, red wine vinegar, dried oregano, salt, and pepper to make the dressing.
3. Pour the dressing over the salad ingredients and toss until evenly coated.
4. Divide the Greek salad mixture among serving cups or small plates.
5. Garnish with fresh parsley, if desired.
6. Serve immediately as an appetizer or side dish.

NUTRITIONAL INFORMATION (PER SERVING):

Calories: 120 | Carbs: 5g | Fiber: 2g | Net Carbs: 3g

Protein: 2g | Fats: 10g

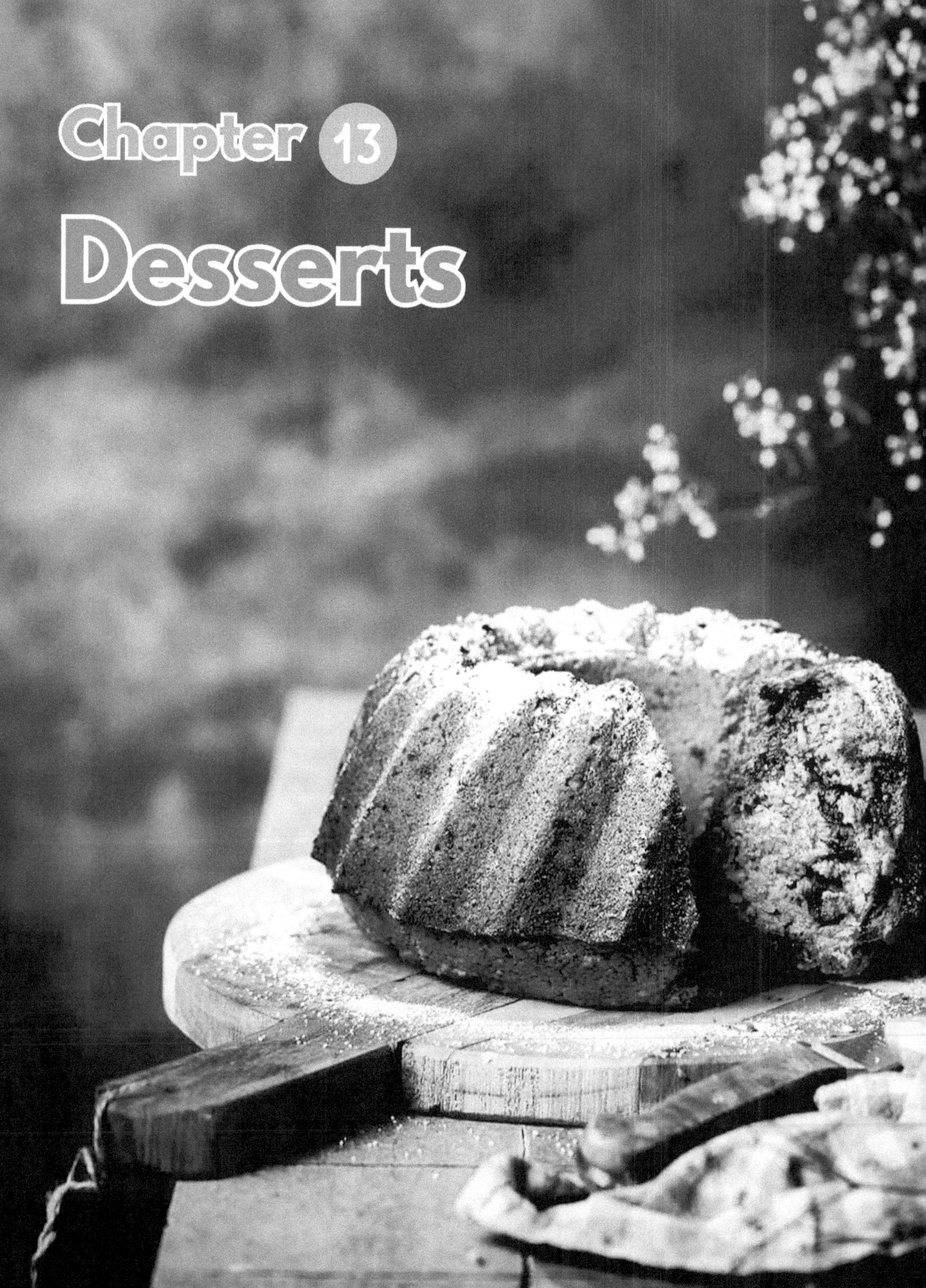

Chapter 13
Desserts

Coconut Flour Chocolate Chip Cookies

Prep Time: 15 Minutes | **Cook Time:** 10 Minutes |
Serves: 4

INGREDIENTS:

- 1/2 cup coconut flour
- 1/4 cup low-carb sweetener (such as erythritol or stevia)
- 1/4 teaspoon baking powder
- Pinch of salt
- 1/4 cup melted coconut oil
- 2 large eggs
- 1 teaspoon vanilla extract
- 1/4 cup sugar-free chocolate chips

INSTRUCTIONS:

1. Preheat oven to 350°F (175°C) and line a baking sheet with parchment paper.
2. In a mixing bowl, whisk together the coconut flour, low-carb sweetener, baking powder, and salt.
3. Add the melted coconut oil, eggs, and vanilla extract to the dry ingredients. Mix until well combined.
4. Fold in the sugar-free chocolate chips.
5. Scoop tablespoon-sized portions of the cookie dough onto the prepared baking sheet, spacing them apart.
6. Flatten each cookie slightly with the back of a spoon.
7. Bake in the preheated oven for 8-10 minutes, or until the cookies are golden brown around the edges.
8. Allow the cookies to cool on the baking sheet for a few minutes before transferring them to a wire rack to cool completely.

NUTRITIONAL INFORMATION (PER SERVING):

Calories: 150 | Carbs: 6g | Fiber: 3g | Net Carbs: 3g
Protein: 4g | Fats: 12g

Avocado Chocolate Mousse

Prep Time: 10 Minutes | **Cook Time:** 0 Minute |
Serves: 4

INGREDIENTS:

- 2 ripe avocados
- 1/4 cup unsweetened cocoa powder
- Pinch of salt
- 1/4 cup low-carb sweetener (such as erythritol or stevia)
- 1 teaspoon vanilla extract
- Optional toppings: whipped cream, sugar-free chocolate shavings, berries

INSTRUCTIONS:

1. Cut the avocados in half, remove the pits, and scoop the flesh into a food processor.
2. Add the unsweetened cocoa powder, low-carb sweetener, vanilla extract, and a pinch of salt to the food processor.
3. Blend until smooth and creamy, scraping down the sides as needed.
4. Taste and adjust sweetness if necessary by adding more sweetener.
5. Divide the avocado chocolate mousse among serving dishes.
6. Chill in the refrigerator for at least 30 minutes before serving.
7. Serve with optional toppings like whipped cream, sugar-free chocolate shavings, or berries.

NUTRITIONAL INFORMATION (PER SERVING):

Calories: 180 | Carbs: 8g | Fiber: 5g | Net Carbs: 3g
Protein: 2g | Fats: 16g

Almond Flour Carrot Cake

Prep Time: 20 Minutes | **Cook Time:** 30 Minutes |
Serves: 8

INGREDIENTS:

- 2 cups almond flour
- 1/2 cup low-carb sweetener (such as erythritol or stevia)
- 1 teaspoon baking powder
- 1 teaspoon ground cinnamon
- 1/4 teaspoon ground nutmeg
- Pinch of salt
- 1/2 cup melted coconut oil
- 3 large eggs
- 1 teaspoon vanilla extract
- 1 cup grated carrots
- 1/2 cup chopped walnuts (optional)
- Cream cheese frosting (optional)

1. Preheat your oven to 350°F (175°C). Grease an 8-inch round cake pan and line the bottom with parchment paper.
2. In a large bowl, whisk together the almond flour, low-carb sweetener, baking powder, ground cinnamon, ground nutmeg, and a pinch of salt.
3. In a separate bowl, whisk together the melted coconut oil, eggs, and vanilla extract.
4. Add the wet ingredients to the dry ingredients and mix until well combined.
5. Fold in the grated carrots and chopped walnuts, if using.
6. Pour the batter into the prepared cake pan and spread it out evenly.
7. Bake in the preheated oven for 25-30 minutes, or until a toothpick inserted into the center comes out clean.
8. Allow the cake to cool in the pan for 10 minutes, then transfer it to a wire rack to cool completely.
9. Once cooled, frost the cake with cream cheese frosting, if desired.
10. Slice and serve.

NUTRITIONAL INFORMATION (PER SERVING):

Calories: 280 | Carbs: 7g | Fiber: 3g | Net Carbs: 4g
Protein: 8g | Fats: 24g

Sponge Cake

Prep Time: 15 Minutes | **Cook Time:** 20 Minutes | **Serves:** 8

INGREDIENTS:

- 6 large eggs
- 1/2 cup low-carb sweetener (such as erythritol or stevia)
- 1 teaspoon vanilla extract
- 1/2 cup almond flour
- 1/4 cup coconut flour
- 1 teaspoon baking powder
- Pinch of salt

INSTRUCTIONS:

1. Start by preheating your oven to 350°F (175°C). Grease an 8-inch square cake pan and line the bottom with parchment paper.
2. In a large mixing bowl, beat the eggs and low-carb sweetener together until pale and fluffy.
3. Add the vanilla extract and mix until combined.

4. In a separate bowl, whisk together the almond flour, coconut flour, baking powder, and a pinch of salt.
5. Gradually add the dry ingredients to the egg mixture, folding gently until just combined.
6. Pour the batter into the prepared cake pan and spread it out evenly.
7. Bake in the preheated oven for 18-20 minutes, or until the cake is golden brown and springs back when lightly touched.
8. Allow the cake to cool in the pan for 10 minutes, then transfer it to a wire rack to cool completely.
9. Once cooled, slice and serve.

NUTRITIONAL INFORMATION (PER SERVING):

Calories: 120 | Carbs: 5g | Fiber: 2g | Net Carbs: 3g
Protein: 6g | Fats: 8g

Raspberry Lemon Cheesecake Bars

Prep Time: 20 Minutes | **Cook Time:** 45 Minutes | **Serves:** 12

INGREDIENTS:

Crust:

- 1 1/2 cups almond flour
- 1/4 cup low-carb sweetener (such as erythritol or stevia)
- 1/4 teaspoon salt
- 1/4 cup melted coconut oil

Raspberry Swirl:

- 1/2 cup fresh or frozen raspberries
- 2 tablespoons low-carb sweetener (such as erythritol or stevia)
- 1 tablespoon lemon juice

Cheesecake Filling:

- 16 oz cream cheese, softened
- 1/2 cup low-carb sweetener (such as erythritol or stevia)
- 2 large eggs
- 1 teaspoon vanilla extract
- Zest of 1 lemon
- Juice of 1 lemon

INSTRUCTIONS:

1. Preheat your oven to 325°F (160°C). Grease an 8x8-inch baking dish and line it with parchment paper,

leaving some overhang on the sides for easy removal.

2. In a mixing bowl, combine the almond flour, low-carb sweetener, and salt for the crust. Stir in the melted coconut oil until the mixture resembles coarse crumbs.
3. Press the crust mixture evenly into the bottom of the prepared baking dish.
4. Bake the crust in the preheated oven for 10 minutes, then remove it and set it aside.
5. In another mixing bowl, beat the softened cream cheese and low-carb sweetener for the cheesecake filling until smooth and creamy.
6. Add the eggs, one at a time, beating well after each addition.
7. Stir in the vanilla extract, lemon zest, and lemon juice until well combined.
8. Pour the cheesecake filling over the baked crust in the baking dish, spreading it out evenly.
9. In a small saucepan, combine the raspberries, low-carb sweetener, and lemon juice for the raspberry swirl. Cook over medium heat, stirring occasionally, until the raspberries break down and the mixture thickens slightly, about 5 minutes. Remove from heat and strain through a fine mesh sieve to remove the seeds, pressing down with a spoon to extract all the liquid.
10. Spoon dollops of the raspberry sauce over the cheesecake filling, then use a knife or toothpick to swirl it into the cheesecake batter.
11. Bake the cheesecake in the preheated oven for 35-40 minutes, or until the edges are set and the center is just slightly jiggly.
12. Allow the cheesecake to cool completely at room temperature, then refrigerate for at least 3-4 hours or overnight before slicing into bars.
13. Once chilled, slice the cheesecake into bars and serve.

NUTRITIONAL INFORMATION (PER SERVING):

Calories: 180 | Carbs: 5g | Fiber: 2g | Net Carbs: 3g
Protein: 6g | Fats: 14g

No-Bake Peanut Butter Balls

Prep Time: 15 Minutes | **Chill Time:** 30 Minutes |
Serves: 12

INGREDIENTS:

- 1 cup natural peanut butter (unsweetened)
- 1/4 cup unsweetened shredded coconut
- 1/4 cup low-carb sweetener (such as erythritol or stevia)
- 1/4 cup coconut flour
- 1 teaspoon vanilla extract
- Pinch of salt
- 2-3 tablespoons unsweetened almond milk (if needed)
- Additional unsweetened shredded coconut for rolling (optional)

INSTRUCTIONS:

1. In a mixing bowl, combine the natural peanut butter, low-carb sweetener, coconut flour, unsweetened shredded coconut, vanilla extract, and a pinch of salt.
2. Mix until well combined. If the mixture is too dry, add unsweetened almond milk, 1 tablespoon at a time, until the mixture holds together.
3. Roll the mixture into tablespoon-sized balls using your hands.
4. If desired, roll the balls in additional unsweetened shredded coconut to coat.
5. Place the peanut butter balls on a baking sheet lined with parchment paper.
6. Chill in the refrigerator for at least 30 minutes before serving.

NUTRITIONAL INFORMATION (PER SERVING):

Calories: 130 | Carbs: 5g | Fiber: 2g | Net Carbs: 3g
Protein: 5g | Fats: 10g

Strawberry and Mascarpone Tart

Prep Time: 20 Minutes | **Cook Time:** 10 Minutes |
Serves: 8

INGREDIENTS:

Crust:

- 1 1/2 cups almond flour
- 1/4 cup low-carb sweetener (such as erythritol or stevia)
- 1/4 cup melted coconut oil

Filling:

- 8 oz mascarpone cheese, softened
- 1/4 cup low-carb sweetener (such as erythritol or stevia)
- 1 teaspoon vanilla extract
- 1 cup sliced strawberries

INSTRUCTIONS:

1. Preheat your oven to 350°F (175°C). Grease a 9-inch tart pan with a removable bottom.
2. In a mixing bowl, combine the almond flour, low-carb sweetener, and melted coconut oil for the crust.
3. Press the crust mixture evenly into the bottom and up the sides of the tart pan.
4. Bake the crust in the preheated oven for 8-10 minutes, or until lightly golden brown.
5. Remove the crust from the oven and let it cool completely.
6. In another mixing bowl, beat the softened mascarpone cheese, low-carb sweetener, and vanilla extract until smooth and creamy.
7. Spread the mascarpone filling evenly over the cooled crust.
8. Arrange the sliced strawberries on top of the mascarpone filling.
9. Chill the tart in the refrigerator for at least 2 hours before serving.

NUTRITIONAL INFORMATION (PER SERVING):

Calories: 280 | Carbs: 6g | Fiber: 2g | Net Carbs: 4g
Protein: 6g | Fats: 26g

Pineapple Pear Medley

Prep Time: 10 Minutes | **Cook Time:** 0 Minute |
Serves: 4

INGREDIENTS:

* 1 cup diced pineapple
* 1 cup diced pear
* 2 tablespoons fresh lime juice
* 1 tablespoon chopped fresh mint leaves
* 1 tablespoon low-carb sweetener (such as erythritol or stevia) (optional)
* Unsweetened coconut flakes for garnish (optional)

INSTRUCTIONS:

1. In a serving bowl, combine the diced pineapple and diced pear.
2. Drizzle the fresh lime juice over the fruit and toss to coat.
3. If desired, sprinkle the chopped fresh mint leaves and low-carb sweetener over the fruit and toss again.
4. Garnish with unsweetened coconut flakes, if desired.

5. Serve immediately or chill in the refrigerator before serving.

NUTRITIONAL INFORMATION (PER SERVING):

Calories: 70 | Carbs: 18g | Fiber: 3g | Net Carbs: 15g
Protein: 1g | Fats: 0g

Flourless Chocolate Cake

Prep Time: 15 Minutes | **Cook Time:** 25 Minutes |
Serves: 8

INGREDIENTS:

* 8 oz (225g) unsweetened chocolate, chopped
* 3/4 cup (170g) unsalted butter
* 1 cup (200g) low-carb sweetener (such as erythritol or stevia)
* 4 large eggs
* 1 teaspoon vanilla extract
* Pinch of salt
* Whipped cream or berries for serving (optional)

INSTRUCTIONS:

1. Preheat your oven to 350°F (175°C). Grease an 8-inch round cake pan and line the bottom with parchment paper.
2. In a heatproof bowl set over a pot of simmering water, melt the chopped chocolate and unsalted butter together, stirring until smooth. Remove from heat and let cool slightly.
3. In a separate mixing bowl, whisk together the low-carb sweetener, eggs, vanilla extract, and a pinch of salt until well combined.
4. Gradually pour the melted chocolate mixture into the egg mixture, whisking continuously until smooth.
5. Pour the batter into the prepared cake pan and spread it out evenly.
6. Bake in the preheated oven for 20-25 minutes, or until the edges are set and the center is slightly jiggly.
7. Remove from the oven and let the cake cool completely in the pan on a wire rack.
8. Once cooled, run a knife around the edges of the cake to loosen it from the pan. Invert the cake onto a serving plate.
9. Serve slices of the flourless chocolate cake with whipped cream or berries, if desired.

Calories: 300 | Carbs: 5g | Fiber: 3g | Net Carbs: 2g

Protein: 6g | Fats: 28g

Keto Blueberry Muffins

Prep Time: 10 Minutes | **Cook Time:** 25 Minutes
Serves: 12

INGREDIENTS:

- ❖ 2 cups almond flour
- ❖ 1/3 cup low-carb sweetener (such as erythritol or stevia)
- ❖ 1 teaspoon baking powder
- ❖ 1/4 cup melted coconut oil
- ❖ 1/4 teaspoon salt
- ❖ 3 large eggs
- ❖ 1/4 cup unsweetened almond milk
- ❖ 1 teaspoon vanilla extract
- ❖ 1 cup fresh or frozen blueberries

INSTRUCTIONS:

1. Preheat your oven to 350°F (175°C). Line a muffin tin with paper liners or grease well.
2. In a large mixing bowl, whisk together the almond flour, low-carb sweetener, baking powder, and salt.
3. In a separate bowl, beat the eggs, melted coconut oil, almond milk, and vanilla extract until well combined.
4. Gradually add the wet ingredients to the dry ingredients, stirring until just combined.
5. Gently fold in the blueberries.
6. Divide the batter evenly among the prepared muffin cups.
7. Bake in the preheated oven for 20-25 minutes, or until golden brown and a toothpick inserted into the center comes out clean.
8. Remove from the oven and let the muffins cool in the pan for 5 minutes before transferring them to a wire rack to cool completely.

NUTRITIONAL INFORMATION (PER SERVING):

Calories: 150 | Carbs: 5g | Fiber: 2g | Net Carbs: 3g

Protein: 5g | Fats: 12g

Lemon and Poppy Seed Loaf

Prep Time: 15 Minutes | **Cook Time:** 45 Minutes
Serves: 10

INGREDIENTS:

- ❖ 2 cups almond flour
- ❖ 1/3 cup low-carb sweetener (such as erythritol or stevia)
- ❖ 1 teaspoon baking powder
- ❖ 1/4 teaspoon salt
- ❖ Zest of 2 lemons
- ❖ 1/4 cup fresh lemon juice
- ❖ 1/4 cup melted coconut oil
- ❖ 3 large eggs
- ❖ 1 teaspoon vanilla extract
- ❖ 1 tablespoon poppy seeds

INSTRUCTIONS:

1. Preheat your oven to 350°F (175°C). Grease a loaf pan and line the bottom with parchment paper.
2. In a large mixing bowl, whisk together the almond flour, low-carb sweetener, baking powder, salt, and lemon zest.
3. In a separate bowl, whisk together the fresh lemon juice, melted coconut oil, eggs, and vanilla extract.
4. Gradually add the wet ingredients to the dry ingredients, stirring until just combined.
5. Fold in the poppy seeds.
6. Pour the batter into the prepared loaf pan and spread it out evenly.
7. Bake in the preheated oven for 40-45 minutes, or until golden brown and a toothpick inserted into the center comes out clean.
8. Remove from the oven and let the loaf cool in the pan for 10 minutes before transferring it to a wire rack to cool completely.

NUTRITIONAL INFORMATION (PER SERVING):

Calories: 180 | Carbs: 5g | Fiber: 2g | Net Carbs: 3g

Protein: 6g | Fats: 14g

Chocolate Avocado Pudding

Prep Time: 10 Minutes | **Cook Time:** 0 Minute
Serves: 4

- 2 ripe avocados
- 1/4 cup unsweetened cocoa powder
- 1/4 cup low-carb sweetener (such as erythritol or stevia)
- 1 teaspoon vanilla extract
- Pinch of salt
- 1/4 cup unsweetened almond milk (or any milk of choice)
- Optional toppings: whipped cream, berries, nuts

INSTRUCTIONS:

1. Peel and pit the avocados, then scoop the flesh into a food processor.
2. Add the cocoa powder, low-carb sweetener, vanilla extract, salt, and almond milk to the food processor.
3. Blend until smooth and creamy, scraping down the sides as needed to ensure everything is well incorporated.
4. Taste the pudding and adjust sweetness if necessary by adding more sweetener.
5. Divide the chocolate avocado pudding among serving dishes.
6. Chill in the refrigerator for at least 30 minutes before serving.
7. Serve with optional toppings like whipped cream, berries, or nuts.

NUTRITIONAL INFORMATION (PER SERVING):

Calories: 150 | Carbs: 8g | Fiber: 5g | Net Carbs: 3g
Protein: 2g | Fats: 3g

Vanilla Bean Panna Cotta

Prep Time: 15 Minutes | **Cook Time:** 5 Minutes | **Chill Time:** 4 Hours | **Serves:** 4

INGREDIENTS:

- 1 cup heavy cream
- 1 cup unsweetened almond milk (or any milk of choice)
- 1/4 cup low-carb sweetener (such as erythritol or stevia)
- 1 vanilla bean pod, split lengthwise and seeds scraped out (or 1 teaspoon vanilla extract)
- 2 teaspoons unflavored gelatin powder
- 2 tablespoons cold water

INSTRUCTIONS:

1. In a saucepan, combine the heavy cream, almond milk, low-carb sweetener, and scraped vanilla bean seeds (or vanilla extract). Heat over medium heat, stirring occasionally, until the mixture is steaming but not boiling. Remove from heat.
2. In a small bowl, sprinkle the gelatin powder over the cold water and let it sit for a minute to bloom.
3. Once bloomed, whisk the gelatin mixture into the warm cream mixture until completely dissolved.
4. Strain the mixture through a fine mesh sieve to remove any lumps or vanilla bean remnants.
5. Divide the mixture among serving glasses or ramekins.
6. Chill in the refrigerator for at least 4 hours, or until set.
7. Serve the vanilla bean panna cotta chilled, garnished with fresh berries or mint leaves if desired.

NUTRITIONAL INFORMATION (PER SERVING):

Calories: 250 | Carbs: 5g | Fiber: 0g | Net Carbs: 5g
Protein: 2g | Fats: 25g

Mixed Berry Crumble with Almond

Prep Time: 15 Minutes | **Cook Time:** 30 Minutes | **Serves:** 6

INGREDIENTS:

Filling:
- 4 cups mixed berries (such as strawberries, blueberries, raspberries, blackberries)
- 2 tablespoons low-carb sweetener (such as erythritol or stevia)
- 1 tablespoon lemon juice
- 1 tablespoon arrowroot powder or cornstarch (optional, for thickening)

Topping:
- 1 cup almond flour
- 1/4 cup low-carb sweetener (such as erythritol or stevia)
- 1/4 cup chopped almonds
- 1/4 cup unsalted butter, melted
- 1 teaspoon ground cinnamon
- Pinch of salt

1. Preheat your oven to 350°F (175°C). Grease a baking dish.
2. In a mixing bowl, toss the mixed berries with low-carb sweetener, lemon juice, and arrowroot powder or cornstarch (if using). Transfer the berry mixture to the prepared baking dish.
3. In another mixing bowl, combine almond flour, low-carb sweetener, chopped almonds, melted butter, cinnamon, and a pinch of salt. Mix until crumbly.
4. Sprinkle the almond topping evenly over the mixed berries in the baking dish.
5. Bake in the preheated oven for 25-30 minutes, or until the topping is golden brown and the berries are bubbling.
6. Remove from the oven and let cool slightly before serving.
7. Serve the mixed berry crumble warm, optionally topped with whipped cream or a dollop of Greek yogurt.

NUTRITIONAL INFORMATION (PER SERVING):

Calories: 220 | Carbs: 10g | Fiber: 4g | Net Carbs: 6g
Protein: 4g | Fats: 18g

Cinnamon Flaxseed Muffins

Prep Time: 10 Minutes | **Cook Time:** 25 Minutes |
Serves: 12

INGREDIENTS:

- 2 cups ground flaxseed meal
- 1/2 cup low-carb sweetener (such as erythritol or stevia)
- 2 teaspoons baking powder
- 1 tablespoon ground cinnamon
- Pinch of salt
- 4 large eggs
- 1/2 cup unsweetened almond milk (or any milk of choice)
- 1/4 cup melted coconut oil
- 1 teaspoon vanilla extract

INSTRUCTIONS:

1. Preheat your oven to 350°F (175°C). Line a muffin tin with paper liners or grease well.
2. In a large mixing bowl, combine the ground flaxseed meal, low-carb sweetener, baking powder, cinnamon, and a pinch of salt.
3. In another bowl, whisk together the eggs, almond milk, melted coconut oil, and vanilla extract until well combined.
4. Gradually add the wet ingredients to the dry ingredients, stirring until just combined.
5. Divide the batter evenly among the prepared muffin cups.
6. Bake in the preheated oven for 20-25 minutes, or until the muffins are golden brown and a toothpick inserted into the center comes out clean.
7. Remove from the oven and let the muffins cool in the pan for 5 minutes before transferring them to a wire rack to cool completely

NUTRITIONAL INFORMATION (PER SERVING):

Calories: 150 | Carbs: 5g | Fiber: 4g | Net Carbs: 1g
Protein: 5g | Fats: 12g

Chocolate Hazelnut Truffles

Prep Time: 20 Minutes | **Chill Time:** 1 Hour |
Serves: 12

INGREDIENTS:

- 1/2 cup hazelnuts, toasted and skins removed
- 1/4 cup unsweetened cocoa powder
- 2 tablespoons low-carb sweetener (such as erythritol or stevia)
- 2 tablespoons coconut oil, melted
- 1 teaspoon vanilla extract
- Pinch of salt
- Additional cocoa powder or chopped hazelnuts for rolling (optional)

INSTRUCTIONS:

1. In a food processor, pulse the toasted hazelnuts until finely ground.
2. Add the cocoa powder, low-carb sweetener, melted coconut oil, vanilla extract, and a pinch of salt to the food processor.
3. Process until the mixture comes together and forms a thick paste.
4. Taste the mixture and adjust sweetness if necessary.
5. Scoop out small portions of the mixture and roll them into balls between your palms.
6. If desired, roll the truffles in additional cocoa powder or chopped hazelnuts for coating.

7. Place the rolled truffles on a baking sheet lined with parchment paper.
8. Chill the truffles in the refrigerator for at least 1 hour before serving.

Calories: 90 | Carbs: 3g | Fiber: 2g | Net Carbs: 1g
Protein: 2g | Fats: 8g

Berry Bubble

Prep Time: 15 Minutes | **Cook Time:** 30 Minutes | **Serves:** 6

INGREDIENTS:

Filling:

*   4 cups mixed berries (such as strawberries, blueberries, raspberries, blackberries)
*   1/4 cup low-carb sweetener (such as erythritol or stevia)
*   1 tablespoon lemon juice
*   1 tablespoon arrowroot powder or cornstarch (optional, for thickening)

Topping:

*   1 cup almond flour
*   1/4 cup low-carb sweetener (such as erythritol or stevia)
*   1/4 cup chopped almonds
*   1/4 cup unsalted

INSTRUCTIONS:

1. Preheat your oven to 350°F (175°C). Grease a baking dish.
2. In a mixing bowl, toss the mixed berries with low-carb sweetener, lemon juice, and arrowroot powder or cornstarch (if using). Transfer the berry mixture to the prepared baking dish.
3. In another mixing bowl, combine almond flour, low-carb sweetener, chopped almonds, melted butter, cinnamon, and a pinch of salt. Mix until crumbly.
4. Sprinkle the almond topping evenly over the mixed berries in the baking dish.
5. Bake in the preheated oven for 25-30 minutes, or until the topping is golden brown and the berries are bubbling.
6. Remove from the oven and let cool slightly before serving.

7. Serve the berry bubble warm, optionally topped with whipped cream or a dollop of Greek yogurt.

Calories: 220 | Carbs: 10g | Fiber: 4g | Net Carbs: 6g
Protein: 4g | Fats: 18g

Orange Almond Cake

Prep Time: 15 Minutes | **Cook Time:** 35 Minutes | **Serves:** 8

INGREDIENTS:

*   1 1/2 cups almond flour
*   1/2 cup low-carb sweetener (such as erythritol or stevia)
*   1 teaspoon baking powder
*   1/4 teaspoon salt
*   3 large eggs
*   1/4 cup unsalted butter, melted
*   1/4 cup unsweetened almond milk (or any milk of choice)
*   Zest of 1 orange
*   Juice of 1 orange
*   1 teaspoon vanilla extract

INSTRUCTIONS:

1. Start by preheating your oven to 350°F (175°C). Grease a cake pan and line the bottom with parchment paper.
2. In a large mixing bowl, whisk together the almond flour, low-carb sweetener, baking powder, and salt.
3. In another bowl, beat the eggs, melted butter, almond milk, orange zest, orange juice, and vanilla extract until well combined.
4. Gradually add the wet ingredients to the dry ingredients, stirring until just combined.
5. Pour the batter into the prepared cake pan and spread it out evenly.
6. Bake in the preheated oven for 30-35 minutes, or until golden brown and a toothpick inserted into the center comes out clean.
7. Remove from the oven and let the cake cool in the pan for 10 minutes before transferring it to a wire rack to cool completely.

Calories: 200 | Carbs: 5g | Fiber: 2g | Net Carbs: 3g
Protein: 6g | Fats: 16g

Prep Time: 10 Minutes | **Cook Time:** 40 Minutes | **Chill Time:** 2 Hours | **Serves:** 6

INGREDIENTS:

- 1 cup canned pumpkin puree
- 1/2 cup heavy cream
- 1/2 cup unsweetened almond milk (or any milk of choice)
- 1/4 cup low-carb sweetener (such as erythritol or stevia)
- 2 large eggs
- 1 teaspoon vanilla extract
- 1 teaspoon ground cinnamon
- 1/2 teaspoon ground ginger
- 1/4 teaspoon ground nutmeg
- Pinch of salt
- Whipped cream for serving (optional)

INSTRUCTIONS:

1. Preheat your oven to 325°F (160°C). Grease 6 ramekins or custard cups.
2. In a mixing bowl, whisk together the pumpkin puree, heavy cream, almond milk, low-carb sweetener, eggs, vanilla extract, spices, and salt until well combined.
3. Pour the mixture into the prepared ramekins.
4. Place the ramekins in a baking dish and fill the dish with hot water until it reaches halfway up the sides of the ramekins.
5. Bake in the preheated oven for 35-40 minutes, or until the custards are set around the edges but still slightly jiggly in the center.
6. Remove from the oven and let the custards cool in the water bath for 10 minutes before transferring them to a wire rack to cool completely.
7. Chill the custards in the refrigerator for at least 2 hours before serving.
8. Serve the pumpkin spice custards chilled, optionally topped with whipped cream.

NUTRITIONAL INFORMATION (PER SERVING):

Calories: 150 | Carbs: 6g | Fiber: 2g | Net Carbs: 4g
Protein: 4g | Fats: 12g

Low-Carb Lemon Curd Tartlets

Prep Time: 20 Minutes | **Cook Time:** 15 Minutes | **Chill Time:** 2 Hours | **Serves:** 12

INGREDIENTS:

Crust:
- 1 1/2 cups almond flour
- 1/4 cup low-carb sweetener (such as erythritol or stevia)
- 1/4 cup unsalted butter, melted
- 1 teaspoon vanilla extract

Lemon Curd:
- 3 large eggs
- 1/2 cup fresh lemon juice
- Zest of 2 lemons
- 1/3 cup low-carb sweetener (such as erythritol or stevia)
- 1/4 cup unsalted butter, cubed

INSTRUCTIONS:

1. Preheat your oven to 350°F (175°C). Grease a muffin tin or tartlet pans.
2. In a mixing bowl, combine almond flour, low-carb sweetener, melted butter, and vanilla extract until a dough forms.
3. Divide the dough into 12 equal portions and press each portion into the bottom and up the sides of the prepared muffin tin or tartlet pans.
4. Prick the bottom of the crusts with a fork and bake in the preheated oven for 10-12 minutes, or until lightly golden brown.
5. While the crusts are baking, prepare the lemon curd. In a heatproof bowl set over a pot of simmering water, whisk together the eggs, lemon juice, lemon zest, and low-carb sweetener until smooth.
6. Add the cubed butter to the bowl and continue whisking until the mixture thickens enough to coat the back of a spoon.
7. Remove from heat and strain the lemon curd through a fine mesh sieve to remove any lumps.
8. Once the crusts are baked, pour the lemon curd into each crust.
9. Chill the tartlets in the refrigerator for at least 2 hours, or until the lemon curd is set.
10. Serve the low-carb lemon curd tartlets chilled.

NUTRITIONAL INFORMATION (PER SERVING):

Calories: 180 | Carbs: 5g | Fiber: 2g | Net Carbs: 3g
Protein: 4g | Fats: 15g

Keto Chocolate Ice Cream

Prep Time: 10 Minutes | **Chill Time:** 4 Hours | **Serves:** 6

INGREDIENTS:

- 1 cup unsweetened almond milk (or any milk of choice)
- 1/2 cup low-carb sweetener (such as erythritol or stevia)
- 2 cups heavy cream
- 1/4 cup unsweetened cocoa powder
- 1 teaspoon vanilla extract
- Pinch of salt

INSTRUCTIONS:

1. In a mixing bowl, whisk together the heavy cream, almond milk, low-carb sweetener, cocoa powder, vanilla extract, and a pinch of salt until well combined.
2. Pour the mixture into an ice cream maker and churn according to the manufacturer's instructions until it reaches the desired consistency.
3. Transfer the churned ice cream to a freezer-safe container and freeze for at least 4 hours, or until firm.
4. Serve the keto chocolate ice cream scoops in bowls or cones, optionally topped with whipped cream or sugar-free chocolate syrup.

NUTRITIONAL INFORMATION (PER SERVING):

Calories: 250 | Carbs: 5g | Fiber: 2g | Net Carbs: 3g
Protein: 3g | Fats: 25g

Coconut and Almond Bark

Prep Time: 10 Minutes | **Chill Time:** 1 Hour | **Serves:** 8

INGREDIENTS:

- 1 cup unsweetened shredded coconut
- 1/2 cup sliced almonds
- 1/4 cup unsweetened coconut oil, melted
- 2 tablespoons low-carb sweetener (such as erythritol or stevia)
- 1/2 teaspoon vanilla extract
- Pinch of salt

INSTRUCTIONS:

1. Line a baking sheet with parchment paper or a silicone mat.
2. In a mixing bowl, combine the shredded coconut, sliced almonds, melted coconut oil, low-carb sweetener, vanilla extract, and a pinch of salt. Mix until well combined.
3. Spread the mixture evenly onto the prepared baking sheet.
4. Place the baking sheet in the refrigerator and chill for at least 1 hour, or until the bark is firm.
5. Once chilled, break the coconut and almond bark into pieces.
6. Store the bark in an airtight container in the refrigerator until ready to serve.

NUTRITIONAL INFORMATION (PER SERVING):

Calories: 160 | Carbs: 4g | Fiber: 2g | Net Carbs: 2g
Protein: 3g | Fats: 15g

Peanut Butter and Jelly Thumbprint

Prep Time: 15 Minutes | **Cook Time:** 12 Minutes | **Serves:** 12

INGREDIENTS:

- 1/4 cup low-carb sweetener (such as erythritol or stevia)
- 1/4 cup unsalted butter, softened
- 1/4 cup unsweetened peanut butter
- 1 cup almond flour
- 1 large egg
- 1/2 teaspoon vanilla extract
- 2 tablespoons sugar-free raspberry or strawberry jam

INSTRUCTIONS:

1. Preheat your oven to 350°F (175°C). Line a baking sheet with parchment paper.
2. In a mixing bowl, cream together the almond flour, low-carb sweetener, softened butter, peanut butter, egg, and vanilla extract until a dough forms.
3. Roll the dough into 12 equal-sized balls and place them on the prepared baking sheet.
4. Use your thumb or the back of a spoon to make an indentation in the center of each cookie.
5. Fill each indentation with about 1/2 teaspoon of sugar-free jam.
6. Bake in the preheated oven for 10-12 minutes, or until

the cookies are golden brown around the edges.

7. Remove from the oven and let the cookies cool on the baking sheet for 5 minutes before transferring them to a wire rack to cool completely.

Calories: 150 | Carbs: 4g | Fiber: 2g | Net Carbs: 2g

Protein: 4g | Fats: 12g

Walnut Macaroons

Prep Time: 15 Minutes | **Cook Time:** 15 Minutes | **Serves:** 12

INGREDIENTS:

- ❖ 2 cups finely ground walnuts
- ❖ 1/4 cup low-carb sweetener (such as erythritol or stevia)
- ❖ 2 large egg whites
- ❖ 1 teaspoon vanilla extract
- ❖ Pinch of salt

INSTRUCTIONS:

1. Start by preheating your oven to 350°F (175°C). Line a baking sheet with parchment paper.
2. In a mixing bowl, combine the finely ground walnuts, low-carb sweetener, egg whites, vanilla extract, and a pinch of salt. Mix until well combined.
3. Scoop tablespoon-sized portions of the mixture onto the prepared baking sheet, spacing them apart.
4. Use your fingers or the back of a spoon to shape the mixture into small mounds or rounds.
5. Bake in the preheated oven for 12-15 minutes, or until the macaroons are lightly golden brown around the edges.
6. Remove from the oven and let the macaroons cool on the baking sheet for 5 minutes before transferring them to a wire rack to cool completely.

NUTRITIONAL INFORMATION (PER SERVING):

Calories: 120 | Carbs: 3g | Fiber: 1g | Net Carbs: 2g

Protein: 3g | Fats: 10g

Baked Ricotta with Lemon and Thyme

Prep Time: 10 Minutes | **Cook Time:** 25 Minutes | **Serves:** 4

INGREDIENTS:

- ❖ 1 cup ricotta cheese
- ❖ Zest of 1 lemon
- ❖ 1 tablespoon fresh lemon juice
- ❖ Salt and pepper to taste
- ❖ 1 tablespoon fresh thyme leaves (or 1 teaspoon dried thyme)
- ❖ 2 tablespoons grated Parmesan cheese (optional)

INSTRUCTIONS:

1. Preheat your oven to 375°F (190°C).
2. In a mixing bowl, combine the ricotta cheese, lemon zest, lemon juice, thyme leaves, salt, and pepper. Mix until well combined.
3. Transfer the mixture to a small baking dish.
4. If desired, sprinkle grated Parmesan cheese over the top of the ricotta mixture.
5. Bake in the preheated oven for 20-25 minutes, or until the ricotta is set and lightly golden brown on top.
6. Remove from the oven and let it cool for a few minutes before serving.

NUTRITIONAL INFORMATION (PER SERVING):

Calories: 150 | Carbs: 3g | Fiber: 0g | Net Carbs: 3g

Protein: 9g | Fats: 11g

APPENDIX 1: MEASUREMENT CONVERSION CHART

VOLUME EQUIVALENTS (LIQUID)

US Standard	US Standard (Ounces)	Metric (Approximate)
2 tablespoons	1 fl. oz.	30 mL
¼ cup	2 fl. oz.	60 mL
½ cup	4 fl. oz.	120 mL
1 cup	8 fl. oz.	240 mL
1½ cups	12 fl. oz.	355 mL
2 cups or 1 pint	16 fl. oz.	475 mL
4 cups or 1 quart	32 fl. oz.	1 L
1 gallon	128 fl. oz.	4 L

OVEN TEMPERATURES

Fahrenheit (F)	Celsius (C) (Approximate)
250°F	120°C
300°F	150°C
325°F	160°C
350°F	180°C
375°F	190°C
400°F	200°C
425°F	220°C
450°F	230°C

VOLUME EQUIVALENTS (DRY)

US Standard	Metric (Approximate)
⅛ teaspoon	0.5 mL
¼ teaspoon	1 mL
½ teaspoon	2 mL
¾ teaspoon	4 mL
1 teaspoon	5 mL
1 tablespoon	15 mL
¼ cup	59 mL
⅓ cup	79 mL
½ cup	118 mL
⅔ cup	156 mL
¾ cup	177 mL
1 cup	235 mL
2 cups or 1 pint	475 mL
3 cups	700 mL
4 cups or 1 quart	1 L

WEIGHT EQUIVALENTS

US Standard	Metric (Approximate)
½ ounce	15 g
1 ounce	30 g
2 ounces	60 g
4 ounces	115 g
8 ounces	225 g
12 ounces	340 g
16 ounces or 1 pound	455 g

APPENDIX 2: THE DIRTY DOZEN AND CLEAN FIFTEEN

The Dirty Dozen and Clean Fifteen

The Environmental Working Group (EWG) provides an annual list known as the Dirty Dozen and Clean 15. These categorize fruits and vegetables based on their pesticide residue level. Food items with the highest residue are listed as the Dirty Dozen, while those with the lowest residue are listed as the Clean 15. By following the list, consumers can minimize pesticide exposure while promoting healthier food choices by choosing conventional options for low-residue produce and prioritizing organic options for high-residue produce, as recommended by the EWG.

2023 DIRTY DOZEN

1. Strawberries
2. Spinach
3. Kale, Collard & Mustard Greens
4. Peaches
5. Pears
6. Nectarines
7. Apples
8. Grapes
9. Bell & Hot Peppers
10. Cherries
11. Blueberries
12. Green Beans

2023 CLEAN FIFTEEN

1. Avocado
2. Sweet Corn
3. Pineapples
4. Onions
5. Papayas
6. Sweet Peas
7. Asparagus
8. Honeydew Melons
9. Kiwi
10. Cabbage
11. Mushrooms
12. Mangoes
13. Sweet Potatoes
14. Watermelon
15. Carrots

APPENDIX 3: RECIPE INDEX

www.ingramcontent.com/pod-product-compliance
Lightning Source LLC
Chambersburg PA
CBHW080846260726
48660CB00009B/3220